Home Remedies

A House Call
from
The Restaurant Doctor™

BILL MARVIN

Hospitality Masters Press
Gig Harbor, Washington

Cover Design: Ad Graphics, Tulsa, OK
Photo Page 141:   Copyright © Stegner Portraits, Colorado Springs, CO

Library of Congress Catalog Card Number: 99-90855

ISBN 0-9656262-7-X

ATTENTION ASSOCIATIONS AND MULTI-UNIT OPERATORS:
Quantity discounts are available on bulk purchases of this book for
premiums, sales promotions, educational purposes or fund raising.
Custom imprinting or book excerpts can also be created to fit specific
needs.

For more information, please contact our Special Sales Department
Hospitality Masters Press, PO Box 280, Gig Harbor, WA 98335
(800) 767-1055, e-mail: masters@harbornet.com, Fax: (888) 767-1055
Outside the US and Canada, phone (253) 858-9255, Fax: (253) 851-6887.

With thanks to Syd Banks, George Pransky and Robert Kausen for helping me understand the power of a quiet mind.

Home Remedies:
A House Call from The Restaurant Doctor™

CONTENTS

APPENDIX

Introduction

This is some of my best material.

The articles in this book are taken from the first several years of my "Home Remedies" newsletter. What makes it my best stuff is not so much in what each article says – although there are some very powerful ideas in here – but in how the article came to be in the first place.

If you have ever produced a newsletter, you know that the demand to have a flow of fresh ideas can be a debilitating experience. I started the newsletter in January of 1995 and filled it primarily with excerpts from my first books. It was a fairly easy process, but I quickly used up most of the material I had written. Now what?

Richard Bach said, "You teach best what you most need to learn." I teach that when your mind quiets down, you tap into a flow of wisdom that is far deeper than anything you access consciously. My bimonthly "brain drain" had the effect of quieting my mind down – the newsletter would be due and I wouldn't have a clue as to what I was going to write!

Perhaps it is because nature abhors a vacuum, but I found that I was suddenly tapping into fresh insights and was seeing the hospitality business in new ways. It was very exciting!

1

As I became more comfortable with the process, I started to see fresh possibilities everywhere. Each time I went out to eat, anywhere in the country, I would notice something would trigger a whole new train of thought. Or someone would ask a question which would start me looking at what I "knew" from an entirely fresh perspective.

That is really the way most of this came together and why it is more a reflection of the process than of the author. This source is available to anyone who is willing to quiet their mind and simply listen for insights.

Some of the items here have made it into one or another of my previous books. Some may yet find a home in another application. If you have a "Marvin library," please forgive any repetition. If you don't, perhaps a tidbit in here will encourage you to pick up another of my books and explore an idea in more detail. Good ideas are good ideas, wherever you find them.

I hope you will enjoy and profit from the notions in this book. Some will make you smile, some may irritate you, but all should make you rethink what you "know" . . . and that will make all the difference.

> Bill Marvin
> The Restaurant Doctor™
> Gig Harbor, Washington

1

Job One . . . and Job Two

Job One is to make sure that the guests are happy. Until that is happening on a consistent basis, nothing else really matters. But what comes next?

I believe the most appropriate task of management is not to run the joint, but to teach **the staff** how to run the joint! This means that our next most important job is training.

Think about it. If you are doing a job that someone on your staff is capable of doing - and you are not giving it to them to do - that is disrespectful.

If you are doing a job that someone on your staff is capable of **learning** and you are not teaching them, that is also disrespectful. Disrespect will drop the climate of your operation faster than most anything else I know.

Not only is teaching your crew how to do your job a respectful act but it will also free you up to tackle new projects that you never had the time to take on before. You might even decide to spend a little more time watching your kids grow up, getting to know your mate or working on your golf swing!

In order for your crew to develop their skills, they are going to have to learn the ropes sooner or later.

Remember that someone taught y<u>ou</u> how to do all these jobs at some point in your career.

Once you have mastered the skill, pass the responsibility along.

2

Doing What is Right

In his book, **Das Energi,** Paul Williams says:

"Nothing is more important than doing what is right. That is so absurdly obvious that most people pay no attention to it. Most people seem to think that what is obvious is beneath them. They pass up truth in favor of something more intellectually stimulating."

Every day we must make decisions – that is the nature of management. When all of the variables are known, this is a relatively simple process. You look up the situation in your data base (personal memory) and handle it based on what you have learned.

However, in any situation involving people, all of the variables are never known. If you try to deal with people problems by relying on personal experience for the answer, it keeps you stuck in the past.

You can only have a memory of things that have already happened – and everything that you already know is what got you into this mess in the first place! To move forward you must find insights and information that you do not yet have – you need fresh ideas.

You get fresh ideas from listening - to other people and to your own inner voice. To access this channel, clear your mind, get quiet and listen.

Listen without even a clue as to what you are listening for. You will know it when you hear it.

Act on it and it will work.

It isn't always intellectually stimulating . . . but it is always right.

3

Do the Best You Can. . . and You're Dead!

Beware the trap of doing the best you can. The real question to ask is **not** how to get orders out 15% faster or how to make 10% more profit (or even how to give the clichéd 110%).

The real question is what level of performance must you deliver if you are to remain a force in the market and prosper into the next century . . . and doing the best you can will not help you achieve it!

The problem comes from incremental thinking – looking at small levels of improvement from your present position.

This may make sense intellectually, but it is unlikely to give breakthrough performance or protect you from savvy competitors who come into the market playing the game at an entirely different level.

When you can define where you need to be and set aside attachment to any current practices in order to get there, you create tremendous opportunity. Freed from the limitations of present thinking, the "impossible" starts to look probable, perhaps even likely.

7

You and your staff will start having fresh insights that will both delight and amaze you. Since they will be creating the new direction, your crew will start to own it. People do not argue with their own ideas.

You do not know what is possible until you stop doing the best you can and start doing what you need to do.

4

A Point to Ponder

At the CHART (Council of Hotel and Restaurant Trainers) Conference in Washington, DC, I heard an idea that deserves further reflection.

Lee Cockerell, Executive Vice President of Walt Disney World, said:

> **"You can't deliver a higher level of service than you have experienced."**

It's an interesting point. If you haven't seen it, how are you going to model it? How can you even begin to understand what I mean when I try to explain it to you?

What is the highest level of service that **you** regularly experience?

Are you always checking out operations comparable to yours or are you visiting folks who are performing at a higher level?

How can you get better without a clear idea of what better looks like?

What do you suppose is the highest level of service the members of your **staff** have experienced?

9

If you want to see material improvements in guest service, they are going to have to visit restaurants that deliver a higher level of service than yours and get a first-hand experience of what is possible.

What operations in your market might serve as that sort of model for your crew?

What should you be doing to promote (or even subsidize) their learning process in this regard?

. . . just a point to ponder.

5
Of Course We Can!

That is the answer to the question.

Which question, you ask? Very simply, **any** question you get from a guest, most questions that you get from your staff . . . and even the majority of those tricky questions that you ask yourself!

The phrase pays homage to "Coach" Don Smith's credo, "The answer is yes. What's the question?" but it takes the idea a bit farther.

Certainly you want to make your guests happy (which will never happen if you tell them what you **can't** do for them!)

Since your staff will treat your guests the same way you treat your staff, it is not a good precedent to start saying no to them, either.

You probably understand it in the context of guests and staff, but how often do you stop yourself from moving to the next level, either personally or professionally, by just automatically thinking that you cannot do it.

Increase sales by 20%? Of course we can!

Cut turnover by 50%? Of course we can!

Have a life? Of course we can!

The way to accomplish these goals will not always be immediately obvious – in most cases it will not be – but by first applying "the answer" and worrying about the details later, you will be amazed at the possibilities you will suddenly start to see.

Do something different? Of course you can!

6

How About a Job With Real Meaning?

Members of the staff at Walt Disney World are authorized – even encouraged – to take five minutes out of their work day at any time to *do something for their guests that the guests will remember for the rest of their lives!*

Think about that – something people will remember for the rest of their *lives!*

Does that sound like a job with real meaning?

Would your staff be up for it?

What do you think would happen if that notion were a part of the culture of your organization?

Would you think of it as a "Big Hairy Audacious Goal?"

It should be clear to everyone who takes the time to ponder the future that "business as usual" is the recipe for disaster. Doing more of what you've been doing will get you *less* of what you already have, so if it isn't broken, the best move may be to break it!

13

But if things are going to change, who is going to take the initiative to chart the new path?

Are you waiting for the market to tell you what to do? Do you expect that someone on your staff will come up with a new direction for you?

If you are going to create a goal as big as the Disney challenge, it must start with you. The only job you cannot delegate is the vision . . . and vision is also a job with some real meaning!

7
Greed

In the movie "Wall Street," Michael Douglas (as the character Gordon Gecko) rhapsodizes that "greed is good." His logic may have fit the film, but it's dangerous in our business.

So what do I mean by greed?

Greed is a concerted effort to maximize revenue by trying to pry the most money you can from each guest that comes in.

Greed is a one-way flow of cash – to you – with hardly a passing thought of sharing the wealth.

Greed is all about what's in it for you.

Greed comes from insecurity – a belief that there is not enough to go around.

It is interesting that what you obsess about often comes to pass.

When you are running scared, it reflects in the way you run your restaurant which impacts how your guests are treated which, in turn, determines whether they come back or not.

15

Greed will kill your spirit and ultimately it will kill your business.

To maximize income, relax, do a better job than you have to do and trust that if you consistently delight your guests, earn their trust and always work in their best interests, they will support you over competitors who are only out for themselves.

In short, leave some money on the table.

Don't try to get every dollar you can tonight. Rather, show guests a great time at a fair price and leave them a little spare change to visit you again.

8

Who Cares?

I have often said that ours, ultimately, is a one-on-one business.

Certainly, we can create spectacular dining environments, engage in clever marketing and offer deals that leave our competitors struggling to catch up. But in the end, the impression guests have of your restaurant is created by the server at the table at the time of the meal.

My question, then, is, "What is the quality of that interaction?"

In the competitive climate we all face, "good enough" is not good enough to make you a legend. The very tangible intangible – your secret to success – lies with your staff and the extent to which they convey a high level of personal caring to your guests.

When people come to your place, will they come away with the impression that it mattered to anyone what kind of experience they had?

. . . that it mattered to you (as expressed thru your staff) how their meal was prepared and served?

17

. . . that it mattered to you (as demonstrated by your staff) that they had a great time?

To survive and prosper into the next century, guests must know without a doubt, as demonstrated by every member of your staff, that *it matters to me what happens to you!*

9

Don't Confuse Hard Work with Results

I was just called in for a second opinion by a client whose restaurant was not performing at the level that he wanted or needed.

As so often is the case, the problem turned out to be the GM. It was not that the manager was not trying – he was a real "horse" who filled in everywhere to get the work done.

The problem, as one of the staff observed, was that "he is putting his back into it . . . but not his heart!"

The dilemma is common.

Managers typically rise to the job based on their performance – what they can **do** – but once there, are judged on what they can get **done**, a totally different game.

There is always work to be done, but it is usually detrimental to the overall well-being of the operation when too much of that work is being done by the manager.

This is particularly true when doing routine tasks

19

prevents him or her from providing passion, one-on-one coaching, guidance, direction and vision – qualities and skills that will actually move the operation forward.

You do not have to prove to anyone that you are the fastest busser or the best dishwasher. In fact, to do so is often disrespectful to your staff.

Your job is not to run the joint, but to teach your **staff** how to run the joint!

Help them to show you their best by letting them see the size of your heart.

10

Happy New Year

Every January, many people take a look at their lives, see things they don't like and make promises about what they are going to do differently.

How many New Year's resolutions have you made . . . and nothing much ever changes?

Doing more of what you have been doing will actually get you *less* of what you have got!

Things will be different only when your thinking changes – when you see old problems from a different perspective.

So if you truly want to make changes, what are you doing to gain a fresh perspective?

Are you regularly reading books that challenge your ideas of "how things are" or are you just looking for ideas that validate what you already think?

When you attend a trade show (you *are* going to trade shows, aren't you?) are you attending seminars? If so, are you looking for fresh approaches or do you feel like you already know more than any presenter?

21

You may have made it to where you are based on what you **know,** but you will grow and prosper in the future based on what you can **learn!**

If you are truly willing to let yourself become a perpetual student, then this year (and every year thereafter) can be a very happy, **new** year!

11

Get Out of Survival

It occurred to me that the operation of many restaurants is really an exercise in survival.

You plan as best you can, but when the doors open, you go into the survival mode and do whatever it takes to get through the shift.

With luck, there are a few minutes at the end of the day to clean up the mess, catch your breath and get a few hours sleep before getting up in the morning and going back into the survival mode again!

So how can you get out of survival?

The first step is to take a longer view. As I have said many times before, your job is not to run the joint, it is to teach your staff how to run the joint . . . and they will never learn how to do it without making a few mistakes along the way.

(Isn't that really the way you learned?)

Never turn anyone loose until they have been thoroughly coached (they will panic and lock up on you), but once a staff member is up to speed, give them the latitude to exercise their own best

23

judgement, even if that means an error or two along the way.

Accept the fact that your staff will do things differently than the way you would – "different" is not the same as "wrong" by the way – and encourage them to use their own creativity.

They will get more involved in the operation and you will have more time to relax, plan . . . and stay out of survival.

12

. . . and the Truth Shall Set You Free

Staff turnover is a real concern for many operators and most have addressed it in one way or another.

A wise few have seen the revolving door as a wake-up call and have reexamined their management approaches but it seems that many have stayed with business as usual and lamented that "you can't get good people anymore" or "these young kids just don't want to work."

Turnover is a symptom

The reason that most approaches to turnover don't work is that turnover is not the problem. It is just a *symptom* of the problem. The simple truth is that your staff leaves because they do not want to stay! If you can find out where the irritations lie, you can start to do something about them.

If turnover is a worry in your operation, the underlying causes are probably not what you think they are. If you knew the real cause of the problem, you would already be on top of it.

But you are not alone in this predicament; we all have blind spots.

25

The trick lies in getting beyond our thoughts of how we **think** things are or how we **want** them to be and get to the truth about what our workers feel about working for us.

An inexpensive but very effective way to find out what it is **really** like to work in your company (and keep a finger on the pulse of the organization) is to conduct exit interviews whenever a staff member leaves.

Feedback gives insights
Smart operators regularly ask their guests how they could do a better job for them the next time because the feedback, however stinging, will help them improve. Similarly, why not ask departing staff members what changes would make your company a more pleasant place to work?

The problem is that workers are most likely to be leaving because of something that management did, something management allowed to happen, or because management did not listen to them. If people felt the company did not listen to them while they worked there, they probably won't feel like telling you much when they leave. Still, the feedback is essential.

If you want to get to the truth, you should look for someone outside the company who is "safe" to talk to and who will respect the confidentiality of the

26

departing worker. In multi-unit companies, there may be a Personnel Department that can handle this function effectively. Smaller operators, however, often have to find another way.

One possibility might be to retain someone on an "as needed" basis to talk with departing staff members. The most effective interviewer will be someone the staff did not have regular contact with during a typical workday – perhaps a retiree or a former worker who resigned to raise a family. Often these people are not looking for full time work but would welcome a little social contact and a few extra dollars.

The advantage of one-on-one exit interviews is that they are more personal and a skillful interviewer can often get past the departing person's natural defensiveness to uncover the real reasons behind their decision to leave. The downside to it is that not all interviewers are effective and a personal interview requires coordinating schedules between the departing worker and the interviewer.

Blind exit interviews
Another alternative for many independent operators and small chains is to use blind exit questionnaires. These are survey forms given to departing staff members. When the ex-employee completes the form and sends it to a third party, they receive a small monetary reward!

The intermediary protects the confidentiality of the information source, sends the money to the employee and forwards completed questionnaires to the company.

This arrangement can be very cost-effective, especially when compared with the costs of turnover. Certainly it is far cheaper than adding an exit interviewer to your payroll, avoids the schedule coordination required to arrange one-on-one interviews . . . and saves your time.

The only disadvantage of the blind approach is that you lose the ability for follow-up questions and clarification of answers. Still, **any** valid information on what it is really like to work for you will shine some light into the blind spots and start to steer you in the right direction.

I acknowledge that it takes courage to actively ask for the truth like this but then foodservice is not a business for cowards! The feedback you receive will give insights into how people feel about working for you and that can make all the difference (if you take it to heart).

Remember the work climate that causes your staff to want to stay longer is the same environment that causes your guests to want to return more often.

This was excerpted from ***The Foolproof Foodservice Selection System,*** copyright © 1993 by John Wiley & Sons, Inc.

13

Turning the Tables

Q: In a recent seminar, someone asked:
"*How can I get a guest to leave when it's busy and I need to turn the table?*"

A: In my opinion, the short answer to the question is "*You can't*" or more accurately, "*You shouldn't try!*"

Here is my reasoning:

The pressure to turn the tables can often cause an otherwise rational operator to go nuts! Just remember that in the hospitality biz, Job One is still to make sure our guests have a good time. That **has** to be our first concern under all circumstances.

It is always dangerous to focus on the needs of the house over the needs of the guests. When we rush one party off the table to seat another, we risk losing the future patronage of the first group.

If that happens, it will cost far more than we might gain from getting the additional seating a few minutes sooner.

All that having been said, the situation can still drive you crazy! Some operators I know encourage their service staff **not** to suggest desserts on busy nights.

That can help . . . **provided** the guests don't have a craving for dessert. If they wanted something sweet and didn't have a chance to get it, they might leave feeling incomplete and that won't help you.

Some operators withhold service in the hopes that the guests will give up and leave. Insanity! This is cutting off your nose to spite your face because you only create disgruntled diners.

A safer approach
My first restaurant was in San Francisco's financial district and, as you might imagine, lunch is prime time for a downtown restaurant.

To maximize sales, we had to handle all the business we could in the two hours that defined the lunch period. At the same time, we could not afford to alienate anyone because the competition in the area was too fierce.

We faced the table-turning question (big time!) every day and developed an approach that usually worked well for everyone.

Here is what we did: When the guests had finished lunch, many would relax and start chatting over coffee. Rather than automatically refilling the coffee after the meal, the service staff would first ask:

30

"Do you have time for another cup of coffee?"

The mention of "time" typically caused the guests to look at their watches. When they realized the time, they would often pass on more coffee in favor of getting back to work.

We got the table back, the guests felt better-served (and didn't get in trouble with their bosses) and everyone was happy!

This article was included in the book, **50 Proven Ways to Enhance Guest Service,** copyright ©1998 by Hospitality Masters Press.

14

More Basics

Many of you are familiar with my very first book, **Restaurant Basics: Why Guests Don't Come Back and What You Can Do About It** – the only book on customer service written entirely from the guest's point of view. It lists nearly a thousand common practices that can combine to leave your diners disenchanted with their experience and it offers suggestions on how to avoid or correct these snags.

Some are obvious (soiled flatware, hair in the food) and some are more subtle ("How's everything?" wet change,). Well, the list is endless. Here are a few more pet peeves, most observed first-hand, from the 250+ additional irritants I have noted since **Basics** was published.

In the interests of space, I will not discuss the reason these items are problems or offer fixes, but you get the idea . . .

- *Seating guests at a deuce when larger tables are empty and business is slow*

- *Offering only deep-fried appetizers*

- *Offering something (grated cheese, etc.) without having it already in hand*

- *Lining the roll basket with a soiled napkin*

- *Pulling a pen out from behind the ear (or the hair) and handing it to the guest*

- *Asking a guest if they would like ground pepper without first giving them a chance to taste the food*

- *Adding an item to the bill after the check has been presented*

- *Leaving completed comment cards from previous guests on the table*

- *Operating lawn sprinklers in the parking lot during meal hours*

- *Uncertain tone of voice (or mumbling) when addressing guests*

- *"The computer is down" (as an excuse for not providing a service)*

- *Bringing a cheap pen with the credit card slip, especially in an expensive restaurant (in this case, a $350 tab for three came with a 19¢ Bic pen!)*

- *Asking an elderly guest if they qualify for a senior citizen's discount (unless they are alone)*

- *Lighting the candle and putting the spent match in the guest's ashtray*

- *Staff letting friends in the back door and seating them (at the window tables) while other guests wait and watch, locked outside in the cold*

- *Serving iced tea with the lemon wedge floating in the glass*

33

- *"You don't want ____ do you? We ran out five minutes ago!"*

- *Pointing when giving directions (always in poor taste, but in this case the patron was obviously blind!)*

- *Staff members talking to each other across an occupied table*

- *"How are we doing tonight?"*

- *Staff leaning on the wall, counter or table when talking to guests*

- *Doing sidework (like rolling silverware) in sight of the guests*

- *Chairs stacked on tables, cushions on the eating surfaces, to facilitate floor cleaning (next to tables where guests are eating)*

- *Staff licking their fingers (observed in a guest waiting area after a server had cut a piece of cheesecake from a glass display case)*

- *Swabbing the dining room floor with a mop obviously from the restroom*

- *Sweeping the crumbs from the table with a floor broom (actually observed in a fast food restaurant – yikes!)*

This material will be expanded in the book, *More Restaurant Basics: Why Guests Don't Come Back and What You Can Do About It,* copyright © 2000 by Hospitality Masters Press.

15

All I Really Needed to Know I Learned on a Saturday Night!

1. Not all birthdays really are.

2. No dishwasher enjoys classical music.

3. If the valet needs to see you right away, take a gift certificate with you.

4. It's really difficult to make Thousand Island dressing at 8:30pm.

5. If a family is waiting long, you will get to know the children real well.

6. Never give the bus person the keys to your smallwares storeroom.

7. If a guest tells you their dinner was OK . . . it wasn't.

8. Restaurant staff have more car problems than the national average.

9. If the broiler person is down to one chicken, it's too late.

10. Service staff who talk a lot about tips usually don't earn a lot of tips.

11. It is important to unlock the front doors when you open.

12. Never leave your keys in the server station.

13. The safe will never open on the first two tries if you are in a hurry.

35

14. You're never out of baked potatoes for only ten minutes.

15. Only write notes to yourself when no one is watching.

16. Ramekins disappear faster than teaspoons.

17. The kitchen and the bar will always need you at the same time.

18. You really *can* smell coffee burning.

19. It's fun to walk outside for a few minutes every hour or so.

20. Children like more than three crayons to color with.

21. When the table is ready for the party of twelve, you will find they are no longer a party of twelve.

22. A reservation who is 20 minutes late will not see it that way.

23. Always check for a reset button before calling the electrician.

24. When you rush, you will always put sweet and sour in a screwdriver.

25. Always thank your crew for a job well done.

These were taken from a list of 101 sent by Bob Hayes of Chart House. Thanks, Bob!

16
How Rules are Really Made

The odds are that you are living with behavior today that results directly from some long-forgotten incident involving a member of your staff who left your employ years ago. You see, every time you chew out one of your crew, you add a new "rule" to your company's unwritten code of conduct.

Nobody likes to be yelled at, so when it happens, you create a very uncomfortable situation. Since you can count on people to avoid pain, the word will travel fast. Not only will there be an impact on all your current staff, but as new people are hired, your veteran workers will tell them, "Oh yes, and make sure you never . . ." and they won't.

But what was the story behind the flare-up that started this paranoia? It could have been a simple misunderstanding, a harmless difference of opinion or an isolated incident.

Perhaps you were just under stress and overreacted. In the end, the exact circumstances really don't matter. You blew your top about something and the "rule" resulting from that upset will continue to be passed along.

This new "rule" will never show up in your operations manual and it is unlikely that any of your staff will ever discuss it with you. (After all, **you** are the one who so clearly expressed your disapproval, so it is obvious how you feel about it!) Still, the fallout from the incident will influence everyone's behavior for years.

So be careful what you say and how you say it. Be alert for rumors and potential misunderstandings. If you even suspect that something is being taken out of context, address it immediately. If you make a mess, clean it up. If you make a mistake, do what you would want your staff to do if one of **them** goofed – apologize, learn from it and move on.

Better yet, conduct yourself in such a way that your actions cannot be misinterpreted. Model the behavior you want to see from your staff. Don't lose your temper. Listen. Watch your tone of voice. Reward progress instead of punishing lapses. Conduct your counseling sessions in private and never when you are angry. As much as possible, create standards of performance rather than rules.

Expect the best and don't jump to conclusions. It is all a human equation, after all.

This article was included in *There's GOT to Be an Easier Way to Run a Business,* copyright © 1999 by Hospitality Masters Press.

17

It's In the Cards

Do you have business cards?

Of course you do. A business card is the mark of a professional in our society. You would feel less than important if you did not have your own business cards, right?

Why would it be any different for your staff? Are they somehow less important or less professional?

One of the best things I ever did when I opened my first restaurant was to print business cards for my crew. I let them put whatever name they wanted on them. I had a bartender that wanted to be called "Coach Pete." When I gave this kid his Coach Pete cards, it was like I had handed him the keys to a new Ferrari!

Everybody on my staff was thrilled! They were passing cards out to all their friends (perhaps because they had cards and their friends didn't, but so what?) We got a lot of trial visits that we were able to turn into regulars.

Then I got smart and said that a signed business card was good for a glass of wine or a free dessert.

39

Now I admit I was nervous about this policy at first. My concern, of course, was the friends of my crew would be drinking free forever! It just did not happen. Nobody abused the privilege. They appreciated the respect and confidence I showed in them.

I had 50 people out there living their lives, meeting people and inviting them back to the restaurant. Marvelous!

In a highly competitive labor market, having business cards might be the factor that causes someone to decide to work for you over a competitor.

In any labor market, your staff can give a card to the people they meet who impress them with their attitude. You might suggest a comment like, "If you know of someone *like yourself* who might be looking for an opportunity, have them come by and talk with us."

Good people tend to hang out with good people (and dirtballs tend to hang out with dirtballs.) Even if that person is not looking for a job, they may have a friend who is.

Foodservice is a business based on personal connection and having cards makes it easier for everyone on your staff to extend a personal

40

invitation - to potential new guests and to potential new staff members.

And what does this grand gesture cost? Unless you have something really fancy, 500 business cards will cost somewhere around ten bucks, particularly if you order in quantity. This means that if you have 30 people on the staff, it will cost you about $300 to get everyone their own cards!

How much advertising can you buy for $300? How much business do you think you might generate from 15,000 personal impressions?

How much money are you spending on classified ads? How effective do you think it would be to encourage your staff to be on the lookout for good people and to slip them a card?

When I bring this idea up in seminars, there is always someone who says that they have blank cards for their staff and the person just writes their own name on the card.

It could be that a fill-in-the-blanks card is better than nothing . . . but maybe it does more harm than good.

How would you feel if I hired you as the GM of my restaurant, gave you a box of blank cards and told you just to write in your name? Pretty unimportant?

41

Business cards are as much a gesture of respect and an investment in morale as they are a sales-building plan or a recruiting ploy. The good news is that it can accomplish all four! . . . for $10!

I would not print cards for someone until they had been employed long enough to complete the adjustment period. (You might call it probation.) Receiving cards would make it more meaningful to make the regular staff.

Some of you may still be concerned. You are going to print cards for people who end up leaving and then you will be out ten bucks! You will have people leave and they will still give out those free wine cards to people who will then come into your place and spend their money. Get a life!

Find something more important to worry about! Instead of reasons not to do it, I suggest you think of some of the exciting possibilities:

How about offering dinner for four to the staff person who has the most signed cards returned during the month? Finally, a contest where the waiters and the dishwashers can compete on equal terms. (My money is on the dish crew, by the way!)

How about a bonus program for staff who refer new workers to you? Cards only make it easier for your staff to be part of the labor solution . . . and it makes a statement to the people they hand their cards to as well.

People say they want to make their staff feel like they were part of things and in my personal opinion, business cards are the most tangible gesture you can make in that direction.

You have to decide how important your staff is to your success. Once you have figured that out, call the printer!

18

Don't Compete – EXCEL!

Nearly every market I visit is experiencing a major influx of new restaurants. Many are chain operations with deep pockets and smooth formats. Some are independents trying to carve out a niche or pursue a dream.

In either case, operators are spending more and more time worrying about the market, looking over their shoulders, counting cars and trying to outguess the new guys.

When they ask me what they should do, I tell them to stop trying to compete! Competing can be dangerous to your professional survival!

Let me explain:

Have you ever been driving down the road and had a police car behind you? I don't know about you but when that happens to me, I suddenly become fixated on the speedometer and fascinated by the rear view mirror!

In this condition, I pay a lot less attention to where I am going! The closer an eye I keep on the cop, the higher my anxiety level rises.

44

I am definitely not as good a driver when there is a cop behind me!

The same thing applies in the business world.

When your attention is primarily on the competition, it drains vital energy away from your primary focus which should be on making sure you run the best restaurant you can.

An obsession with your competitors can interfere with giving your guests a memorable time!

This article was included in the book, ***There's GOT to Be an Easier Way to Run a Business,*** copyright © 1999 by Hospitality Masters Press.

19
Reducing Overtime

Many operators unwittingly create overtime for themselves just by the way they structure their work weeks.

In most restaurants, the pay week runs from Monday to Sunday. Friday and Saturday are the busiest nights.

If you are heavy on hours by the time you get to Friday you are dead. You cannot reduce labor on the weekend because you need everybody you can find to handle the crowd, so you are forced into scheduling overtime.

The solution is to change your pay week. If your pay week started on Thursday or Friday, you would get your busiest period out of the way in the early part of the week when you have plenty of slack on hours.

If you were over on labor after the weekend, you could more easily trim hours on the slower midweek days without as much risk of reducing the level of service to the guests.

20
Is *THAT* All That's Wrong?

Richard Bach, author of **Jonathan Livingston Seagull,** has a great thought in his book, **Biplane.** Discussing the art of repairing old aircraft, he said:

> *"I learn that the repairing or rebuilding of an airplane, or of a man, doesn't depend upon the condition of the original. It depends on the attitude with which the job is undertaken. The magic phrase, 'Is THAT all that's wrong!' and an attitude to match and the real job of rebuilding is finished."*

Every day, managers face situations that call for fast decisions based on a minimum of hard information. Whether these events are stressful or merely look like one more thing to handle is determined by how you see the issue.

If you grasp what is at the root of the difficulty, it is easy to see what needs to be done to solve the problem. As your understanding of human nature deepens, you will find you can approach every "people problem" in your life with this same clarity.

While this new perspective takes a few days to effectively convey to someone, it is within the reach of everyone. Best of all, it is painless and permanent once you see it.

47

Until we have more time, here are three notions that will help you be more effective when facing routine emergencies:

1. When faced with a difficult situation, don't try to "figure it out" – you will not find the answer in your past experience. Instead, clear your mind and reflect on the situation. This will put you in touch with the insights that will contain your answers. When the next step becomes obvious, take it. If you trust the process, it will work.

2. Understand that there are no "bad" people, only good people who get caught in some unproductive thinking from time to time. Behavior is just a response to the way a person sees their world and that world view changes with their state of mind. Don't focus on a person's behavior, look for what is affecting their thinking.

3. Understand that the job of a leader is not to **have** the answers but to be able to **find** the answers. Do not put additional pressure on yourself by thinking you have to know just what to do in every circumstance. You don't. You can't. Often, an honest "I don't have a clue" will help clear your mind and put you in touch with deeper answers.

You will be a more effective leader when you just relax and lead. Clear your head. There is no real problem, you just **think** there is.

"Oh, is **THAT** all that's wrong?"

48

21

A Shining Example of Service

Good service comes from satisfying your guests. Legendary service comes from delighting your guests by totally exceeding their expectations. Here is an example:

It was an evening in early June – the night of the senior prom. Two lovely young women sat in a restaurant waiting for their dates. The wait stretched on and eventually it became obvious the dates were not coming.

Just another teenage tragedy, right?

In most cases, probably so. But Beth Sayers, manager at Clinkerdagger's Restaurant in Spokane was touched by their plight.

She asked the girls if they would mind being escorted to the prom by two of her waiters she recruited to be Prince Charmings.

She obtained the requisite approvals from the girls' parents. She even got the approval of one waiter's wife, who was thrilled that her Australian-born husband would have a chance to see a slice of typical Americana!

49

The restaurant not only supplied the dates, but paid for the hors d'oeuvres the girls had eaten while they waited. Sayers even gave the waiters money for pictures and other prom expenses.

Commenting to the media, Sayers said "Sure it was a nice thing, but what the girls did was far more courageous. We had the easy part. In the face of embarrassment and humiliation, these girls went to their prom."

Now *that* is legendary service!

Its focus is on what it takes to make the guest happy and does not limit itself to the daily mechanics of running the restaurant.

(By the way, this story made the front page of the second section in the Sunday Seattle Times!)

22
Who ARE You?

Have you ever been shopping, found something you wanted, pulled out your checkbook and had to ask the name of the store?

It is entirely possible for people to stumble into your restaurant by accident, have a marvelous meal and leave unable to recommend you because they never really knew where they were! How many times in your service sequence do you let diners know the name of your restaurant?

Here are a few natural ones:

At the door:
  "Welcome to McKenna's."

At the table:
  "Those onion rings are one of McKenna's most popular items."
  "Have you ever tried McKenna's famous rum raisin pie?"

After dinner:
  "Thank you for coming to McKenna's"

Reinforce your name. Imprint it on cocktail napkins or napkin bands. Put your logo on the glassware, ashtrays and matchbooks, even on the wall.

51

23

Start a Mentor Program

Let's say you agree that yours is a 'people business.' My question to you is, "How can you tell?" What is it about the way you operate that is different from a company which is not a 'people business?'

These were the questions I posed to my friends at Phillips Seafood Restaurants . . . and the way they answered them makes my list of all-time great hospitality ideas!

(For background, Phillips operates eight high volume restaurants in the Washington DC/Baltimore area.)

Phillips held a two-day retreat for their GMs and other key management staff to explore "Phillips in the Year 2000" and determine what the company will look like in the new century.

I was a facilitator for the session. We were looking at the human aspects of the business when someone offered, "Phillips in the Year 2000 is a people company."

This prompted me to ask the questions that opened this article.

You see, it is one thing to say you are a "people company," quite another to actually pull it off! We all need a vision of the future but unless we go the extra mile to figure out how to make it happen, we go nowhere.

Taking up the challenge, the group brain stormed about just what would differentiate a "people company" . . . and their answer is brilliant!

After much discussion, we evolved what we called the mentor program.

Every member of the hourly staff was assigned a mentor whose job was to assure that the staff member received at least 30 minutes of quality one-on-one time every month.

These meetings were not to be training sessions but rather, a chance for give-and-take – where the mentors could really listen, learn, and get to know the employee as a person.

As the consensus developed, you can imagine that several of the managers had trouble with the idea.

Since each of them would have about 30 people to work with, they could not see how they were going to find the time.

Mark Sneed, VP of Operations, neatly clarified the

situation. He said, "If we agree that this is what we are as a company, then this *is* what we are and this *is* what we will do. If you want to continue to be part of this group, you do not have the option of *not* making time!" Point made!

I contacted Mark about six months into the program to see what his experience had been. He said the first few months had been a little rough as folks adjusted to the idea but that without a doubt, it was the best thing they had ever done!

He said that if he tried to discontinue it, he would lose most of their staff and all their managers! They got what they expected – productivity was up, turnover was down, and working relationships had improved across the board.

What they got that they didn't expect was that the level of service had measurably improved. Perhaps because the service staff was receiving one-on-one attention from the managers, they were dealing with the guests one-on-one.

Hospitality is an industry that is built on personal connection. The more we foster that experience internally, the more we will deliver it externally.

I urge you to walk your talk, implement a mentor program of your own and be prepared for miracles!

24

Notions

Here are some notions about common courtesy, common sense and the practical applications of the Golden Rule you might want to think about:

1. If you open it, close it.
2. If you turn it on, turn it off.
3. If you unlock it, lock it.
4. If you make a mess, clean it up.
5. If you break it, repair it.
6. If you can't fix it, call someone who can.
7. If you borrow it, return it.
8. If you use it, take care of it.
9. If you drop it, pick it up.
10. If you move it, put it back when you're done.
11. If it belongs to someone else, get permission.
12. If you don't know how to use it, leave it alone.
13. If it doesn't concern you, stay out of it.
14. If you need help, ask for it.
15. If you say you will do it, do it.
16. If you say you won't do it, don't.
17. If you can help, offer.
18. If you can't help, stay out of the way.
19. If you are confused about what to do, ask.
20. If you know what to do, do it.

This material was excerpted from my Staff Manual. For more information, please call.

25

Have Your Cake and Eat it Too

Background

Few national hotel companies actually **own** the properties they **operate** – they operate under a management contract.

Restaurant management contracts (RMC's) are less common but the fundamentals are the same.

Under an RMC, an operator will take over a property (oftentimes distressed) and attempt to make it profitable. He keeps a percentage of the profits for his efforts and the net proceeds pass through to the owner.

Motivations

The owner is motivated to accept the RMC for the following reasons:

- He recognizes his inability to effectively hire and direct a manager and wants to avoid the responsibilities and problems of daily operations.
- His potential return is higher than if he merely leased or subleased the restaurant to another operator.
- If the operator significantly improves profits, the resale value of the property increases by healthy multiples.

The restaurant management company is also motivated to perform well:

- The higher the profit generated for the owner, the greater the reward to the operator.
- The operator can expand without the need to raise a large amount of investment capital.
- Success in providing profits for the owner reinforces the operator's credibility and ability to expand.

Relationship Between Owner and Operator

Most restaurants have two distinct components:

1. **The Operating Entity** which derives revenues and incurs expenses from the sale of food and beverage, and

2. **The Real Estate Entity** which deals with the land, building, improvements and such related aspects as debt service, property taxes, building insurance and invested equity.

Management contract operators are concerned with the first component and owners with the second.

The operator is only responsible for those revenues and expenses which pertain to the actual operation of the restaurant and over which he has control. If the operator is successful, he will generate income from the operation after management fees which will then flow to the owner.

57

Whether or not the income is sufficient to cover the owner's expenses and expected return on investment is another matter. The operator has no control over how much the owner paid for the property and thus cannot be accountable for the adequacy of the income flow with respect to covering the owner's real estate investment.

It is in the operator's best interests, however, to maximize profitability of the restaurant which in turn maximizes cash flow to the owner.

Management Fee Formula
Generally, management companies are paid a percentage (2-5%) of gross sales, called a Basic Management Fee (BMF) plus a percentage of the operating income (15-25%) called an Incentive Management Fee (IMF).

The BMF covers organizational expenses and rewards the operator for increasing sales. IMF is the reward for delivering profits to the owner. The IMF typically accounts for 60% of the fees paid to a management company.

Pitfalls
As you might expect, there are occasionally disagreements between owners and operators as to what are operating expenses and what costs are ownership expenses.

58

The best solution lies in a clearly worded management agreement which addresses these areas in detail, provides appropriate incentives and safeguards all parties. Ultimately, of course, the measure of "workability" in a management contract is reflected in the level of respect and trust between the owner and operator.

Implications

So what does this mean to you? Well, if you are presently the sole investor in your restaurant, an RMC can let you get your cash out of the business and still retain full operating control.

Real estate investors are typically more patient than those who would invest in the restaurant itself, so they do not require the same levels of return to be satisfied. You (hopefully) have a history of generating a positive cash flow from the property and can show a potential investor a predictable return on their investment.

Expansion

Having money does not make you successful in the restaurant business – the ability to run profitable restaurants does. There are more people with money than people who know how to run profitable restaurants.

An RMC allows you to sell your skill, not your financial statement. This may make it easier for you to expand into additional units without the need to finance the whole deal yourself.

Particularly if you have a good reputation in the community and a healthy history of profitable operations, an RMC gives you a structure to let you use other people's money to take on new projects.

Do you have folks who say "If you ever want to do another project, please keep me in mind?" Now you can take them up on it!

Intrigued?

The RMC is truly a way to have your cake and eat it too! Call me for more information or to order a model RMC that has passed through all the legal hoops. (Your attorney should review it . . . but he or she probably couldn't write it!)

26
Just Say Charge It!

A leading Chicago restaurant charges purchases from some of their major vendors using a credit card that rewards them with frequent flyer miles for the dollars they charge.

The restaurant pays their card balance in full every month, so they avoid any interest charges. But best of all, they use the card to buy enough product and supplies to earn, on average, a free trip a week!

Everybody wins with this arrangement. The vendors improve their cash flow because they are paid at the time of delivery. The restaurant gets free travel to attend food shows, reward the staff . . . or give the owners a break!

I think many purveyors would find a plan like this very workable. Propose the idea to your major suppliers and see what sort of reaction you get. They may never have thought of it.

The point is that you are writing the checks anyway. Why not get a few "free" trips for your efforts?

This article was taken from *50 Proven Ways to Build Restaurant Sales & Profit,* copyright © 1997 by Hospitality Masters Press. This idea was contributed by Jim Laube, CPA.

27

Improve Your Tableside Manner

Here is a great way to recover after you have inadvertently asked an inane question like, "Is everything OK?"

When the guest responds, reflect for a moment then ask,

> ***"What would it take to make things absolutely perfect?"***

Listen to their response, reflect on it for a few seconds and then do your best to accommodate them.

Remember that Job One is to make the guest happy . . . and you don't have to be bad to get better!

You know that every once in a while, someone will quip, "Well, absolutely perfect would be if you paid for dinner tonight."

Every once in a while, you might just say, "Done!" (Do it just because it will be so much fun!)

28

Everybody Needs a Hero

Do you have – or have you ever had – an Employee of the Month program? Is it an outstanding success?

Well-intentioned as they are, I have seen few of these programs that endure for very long or truly accomplish the purpose for which they are intended.

The Problem
The difficulty lies in how to fairly decide who is, in fact, the Employee of the Month.

If you were truly honest, the honor would rotate among a select few staff members. If you attempt to broaden the basis for award, it goes to people who are obviously less deserving and that will ultimately undermine the integrity and meaning of the award.

For example, when I started a "Star of the Month" program at the Olympic Training Center, the first selections were obvious but after six months it got tougher. To get my crew involved, I gave everyone a vote. It was a good theory but the selection process quickly became political.

63

The death knell came when the group said, "Let's give it to Tony. He is a lousy worker but we all like him and he hasn't had much recognition." Tony got the award because I did not want to overrule the wishes of the group but after that, the program became a sham and collapsed.

A Modest Proposal
Let's go back to basics. Why would you want an Employee of the Month program in the first place?

"To recognize excellence," you say.

OK, but excellence at what? (thoughtful silence)

If Job One is making the guest happy (and it is!), then I suggest you reward the person on your staff who goes most outside the routine expectations of their job to make the guest happy – in other words, a Hero!

Situation:
A guest accidently locks their keys in the car. Rather than just calling AAA, the cashier gives her own car to a busser who drives the guest home to get the spare set. These people are Heroes.

Situation:
An elderly female guest finds herself with a flat tire in the parking lot. One of your kitchen crew, coming in to work, volunteers to change the tire for her. He is a Hero.

Situation:

A guest's four-year-old is upset. She wants a peanut butter sandwich and there is not one on the menu. The waitress asks the kitchen what they can do and a cook comes out to talk with the child. They discuss brands, the merits of chunky vs. creamy and the best kinds of jelly. The cook then runs to the grocery store for the needed items. The cook (and the waitress) are both Heroes.

These are clear acts of personal initiative in the interest of exceptional guest service that are easy to identify and reward.

Behavior that gets rewarded tends to be repeated.

Instead of an Employee of the Month, look for a Hero of the Month and watch what starts to happen!

29

Customer in Crisis

In hospitals, the phrase "Code Blue" means that a patient is having a life-threatening emergency. When a Code Blue is sounded, all the resources of the hospital mobilize to save the patient.

We need something similar in the restaurant industry. When a guest arrives in a state of advanced agitation, the entire restaurant should go into action to salvage the evening for the diner . . . or at least to be sure not make it worse.

On a consulting engagement, I picked up a way to do this. The code is "CIC" for Customer in Crisis.

The greeter who recognizes that the guest is irritated tries to seat them quickly and notifies the server that the guest is CIC. The server then knows to be particularly attentive and compassionate.

If the guest is still on the edge, a "CIC" note goes on the food ticket, alerting the kitchen to take extra care to be sure the order is exactly right. (You don't want to mess up the dinner of a customer in crisis!) The same with the bar check. The duty manager is informed. All the resources of the restaurant mobilize to "save" the guest.

30
State of the Union

Be on the lookout for increased union organizing efforts as the new leadership of the AFL-CIO tries to recover the lost prestige and clout of organized labor.

The classic way for a union to make a run at you is to have you hire a few of their "ringers" who work their way into a position of peer leadership and start talking up the union. These people will be so well-qualified that they will be hard to turn down when they apply, particularly considering the tight labor market most operators have to deal with.

How do you identify these folks before they have a chance to undermine your organization?

You cannot ask an applicant about his or her position on unions . . . but you can give them yours. Here is a sample of what you can legally say:

We want to maintain a close working relationship with our staff
We are not anti union. However, regardless of what image it tries to project, a union is a profit-making business that can only get money from its own members.

67

To justify its position, a union must create and maintain a "them and us" relationship between the staff and the company. We do not believe such a polarity exists in our organization and we do not think our staff should pay for any such disruptive force.

We believe the way to achieve the kind of business environment we want is to create a trusting relationship with our crew. In this atmosphere, staff and management can work out difficulties and make decisions together. In this environment, a union is unnecessary and is likely to be destructive to operational flexibility and personal well-being.

We cannot imagine a problem we cannot effectively resolve among ourselves without the need for a self-serving third party.

When you put yourself on record like this, you may find that the ringers feel obligated to defend the idea of unions! (An interesting insight to gain into their ultimate suitability for the job, isn't it?)

At the least, your staff will be clear about your position on the subject and will have a more realistic grasp of what a union really is.

The best defense is a good offense.

31
What's Your Problem?

I know, you don't have problems, you have challenges. You might say they are not problems, they are opportunities.

I acknowledge that it is less paralyzing to think of opportunities rather than problems but whatever the euphemism, you are still left with a problem in drag!

However, problems (challenges, opportunities or whatever) are a daily fact of life and dealing with them seems to define the job of most hospitality managers. So let's take another look at problems with an eye toward reaching a different understanding of what is and what is not really a problem.

Problems
A problem is merely a situation that you don't yet have a handle on.

Think about that for a minute. The only reason you would look at a situation as a problem is that you just cannot quite see how to deal with it. Certainly if you knew how to handle it, you would not be likely to think of it as a problem in the first place – a nuisance, perhaps, but not really a problem.

If you are honest with yourself, you have to admit that virtually all of the situations you face in life, personal or professional, ultimately have a workable solution. So when something looks like a dilemma, all you are really facing is an event where the answer is not yet apparent to you. You know there is a solution, you just have to figure out how and where to find it. So there really is no problem.

Conditions

If you have a situation where there is no possible resolution, you do not have a problem, you have a condition. For example, gravity is not a problem, it is a condition.

Now you can love gravity or you can hate it but you are not going to change it! Because gravity is a condition, you are best advised to just accept it and devote your energies to pursuits more productive than complaining about it.

What other "problems" do you face every day (and waste time getting upset about) that are, in fact, really conditions? Government regulations? Taxes? Business seasonality?

32

Coaching Skills

Our model of management is essentially law enforcement – "Find things that are wrong and fix them!" This is fine if you want to spend your life looking for things that are wrong, but there are more productive ways to lead others.

The model we need to adopt is the coaching model. Coaches look for strengths. They take the talent they have to work with and see how they can develop it to win. Coaches say, "You are doing well in this area, now this is the next thing we need to work on."

Coaching is inside-out education where the players see their own answers. (In contrast, what we saw in school was outside-in education where the right answers were held by the teacher.)

To improve your coaching skills, get good at asking questions. Great coaches ask insightful, probing questions that cause their players to think.

It is hard to get yourself in trouble if you are either asking or answering questions. It is only when you are making statements (preaching or lecturing) that you tread on dangerous ground.

33
Inclusion

Q: *How can I make my staff feel like they are part of things?*

A: *MAKE them part of things!*

You can't make folks feel involved if they aren't!

Ask their opinions before making key decisions (listen – really listen – to what they have to say and consider their ideas seriously before taking any action).

Form staff teams to advise you in key areas (operations, rewards and recognition, training needs and so forth).

Give them the latitude (and the budget) to decorate the restaurant for holidays without having to pass everything by management for approval.

In short, fully tap your human resources!

34

Raising Menu Prices in a Competitive Market

Raising prices is a sensitive issue and with more and more competitors in the market, one that needs to be done with care.

One easy move is to have your prices end in .99 rather than .95. You will make an extra 4¢ margin and your guests will not even perceive the change as a price increase.

The best way to avoid the need for an across-the-board price increase (that will set your guests off!) is to reprint your menu frequently and make minor adjustments each time.

This is easy to do if you are printing your own menus on a laser quality printer (a practice I encourage you to consider if the look fits with your operating style.)

Another idea: take an item (whose price you want to increase) off the menu for a while and run it as a special a few times at the higher price. If you meet no resistance, put it back on the menu at the increased price.

35

Training: It's Not Just for Rookies Anymore!

As an operator, I always felt that my only real job was to learn as much as I could and pass as much as I could along to my staff. If you agree, then training becomes an all-the-time thing, not just a one-time program for new hires.

Most operators do a reasonable job of training new hires (although it is usually limited to task-related skills). Once someone knows their way around the place, however, that is usually the last real training they can count on.

Training is a state of mind, not an event.

What does your day-to-day training look like? Do you make sure that you, your staff and your management learn something new every day?

Do you try to learn from your staff as much as you expect them to learn from you? What have you done today to excel?

How do you expect to move forward without continual training for everyone on the staff?

36

Recycling Restaurants

A few weeks ago, I received the following message on my website forum. There have been several comparable questions posted and I just completed a concept redevelopment project with similar characteristics. It appears that the issues raised here are relevant to a number of people, so I thought the question – and hopefully the answer – would be interesting. Here is the original posting:

"One year ago, I took over a local 65 seat restaurant that I believed to have been popular before its closing two years prior. Given my theory on its popularity, I decided to keep the name. The original unit was Swiss and my first opening menu was an upscale contemporary one. My customer base required a shift from that menu. Six months ago I revised the menu to that of an American Bar and Grill serving burgers, ribs, etc. and am starting to achieve some very slow success.

"My question is this: given the not-so-goodwill from the former owner and the not-so-goodwill from my original attempt, is it wise to now change the name to reflect the new menu and hopefully get back some of the people I've lost? Or should I tough it out? Please let me know what you think!"

75

This is an interesting question without a short answer. Let me offer a story to illustrate what I think you need to do:

When Ground Round (an upscale burger concept in the Northeast) was at its peak, its success spawned the predictable imitators. One such wannabe had three units that were not performing well. He approached Ground Round about buying them. "They are exactly your restaurants," he said.

And they were – perfect clones, right down to the paint colors! Ground Round bought them, cleaned them up, hung out the new sign . . . and nothing much happened. They did some intense local advertising . . . and nothing much happened.

Then they closed them again and put in about $100K each in exterior cosmetic changes. They moved the front door three feet, painted the building, re-landscaped the parking area and made similar cosmetic changes. When they reopened, business boomed!

Before the changes, the public did not see that anything was different. It still looked like the same place so it must be the same place. You may know of a few restaurants that have changed hands every year or two that the locals still call by the building's original name. It is still "The Sportsman" to them, even though it is now called "Capt. Jack's!"

76

You can't count on people to figure it out for themselves. So while you don't need to spend $100K, you need to make the place look obviously different enough that people will get that it is a new game. Much of this is external, but there needs to be some internal cosmetics as well.

It's like hitting them over the head with a 2x4 to get their attention. Once they snap out of automatic and get that it is not the same place warmed over, they can start to shift their thinking. Hanging out a sign reading "under new management" (or even "under new attitude") will not make it!

In my experience, the fastest way to make this shift is to invest in the facelift. Close it, change it, reinvent it and reopen with a bang as if you had sold the place to a new owner. It may cost a little more money but I think it will give you the best chance to get an immediate boost in sales volume.

You can tough it out but it is a harder road to travel. It will take you longer to reach the sales volume you want, if you can ever get there at all. In the meantime you will expend an incredible amount of effort, both physical and psychic.

Economics may ultimately determine which way you must go but this is my take on it, for what it is worth.

37
TCB or TCM?

The question that guests have for your service staff is TCB or TCM? Are you taking care of business . . . or taking care of me?

As a guest, I expect you to take care of business. For lack of a better term, we call it service, but service is a mechanical function. It is about serving from the left, clearing from the right and not spilling wine on the table. Service is about timing; it is about serving hot food hot and cold food cold; it is about handling the credit card properly; it is all procedural. Taking care of business is important and your guests expect that you will do it efficiently and consistently.

Hospitality, on the other hand, is a human equation. It is personal. It is about me taking care of you . . . because it is YOU, not because you are one of the 75 people who will pass through my station tonight. You don't take care of 75 people anyway. You deal with one person at a time in 75 different scenarios.

It is the quality of those individual interactions – the level of hospitality you provide – that determines whether I feel that you really cared about ME and my experience.

78

Servers:

Speaking as a guest, when you are just taking care of business effectively, I will usually give about the tip you expected because I got about what I expected. Taking care of business is worth 10-15%.

However, when I get that you are taking care of ME, when you go beyond the normal parameters of your job to provide me with a delightful dining experience, I will leave you far more than you expect and I will be more anxious to return. Taking care of ME is worth 20-30% . . . or more!

Managers:

Lest you feel these comments don't relate to you as well, be aware that the way you treat your staff is the way they will treat your guests. As a member of your crew, when you give me about what I expect, I will give you back about what you expect. But when I get that you are truly interested in ME, that you are working in MY best interests, that you are really listening when I talk to you and that you are considering what I say before you respond, then I will move mountains for you.

In all areas of human interaction, the response you will get from me depends on whether I feel that you are taking care of me or just taking care of business!

This article was included in the book, *50 Proven Ways to Enhance Guest Service,* ©1998 by Hospitality Masters Press.

79

38

Secrets of Consulting – Part 1

I probably should not let you in on this secret, first because it may be bad form for a consultant to let you know how it is done and second, because you might not believe that it can possibly be this easy to find insightful answers to the complex issues that drive you crazy.

In any event, here is the way it works: Let's say an operator has a problem that he or she just can't get a handle on. They finally give up and call me in to help. I talk with them and get their perspective on the problem, of course, but then I will sit down with their staff and ask the crew what is going on.

The operable question is usually something like, "What's wrong with this chicken outfit?"

Then I "get stupid" and just listen.

I find that while no one person typically has the whole answer, collectively there is a wealth of information to be had merely for the asking . . . and the listening.

So I listen without trying to make any immediate sense from what I hear.

80

Then I make observations of my own, get quiet, reflect on what I have learned and wait for the answer to become apparent.

The insight always comes, it is always right on the money – and it is usually very close to what the staff thought should be done in the first place!

(I warned you that you might not believe consulting could be this easy!)

The process involves having the perspective to be able to see what the puzzle looks like once you've identified the pieces. The service is valuable if the operator doesn't have a relationship with the crew where they can talk (and listen) to each other.

My point is that there are few problems you face that cannot be readily solved by the talent already on your payroll!

So why don't more operators tap this resource?

I suspect it is because they have the notion that the manager's job is to have all the answers and that to ask for other people's opinions – and really consider what they have to say – is somehow admitting incompetence.

As a manager, your job is not to have all the answers – that is impossible. Your job is merely to

81

be able to **find** the answers, wherever they are!

Your staff is always closer to the operating realities of the job than you are and, while they may not know how to solve a problem, they certainly can tell you what is making their lives tough.

So if you have the courage to "get stupid," ask questions and really listen to what you hear, you can become very smart, indeed!

You will do less work, your staff will become more involved, you will be impressed with the talent in your employ . . . and you can save a ton on consulting fees!

39
Beware of Research

As a speaker, I constantly hear people advocating the need for – and the importance of – detailed research to support every statement.

The theory is fine but I caution you to beware (or at least to be wary) of research.

If you did a survey in the year 1491, it would have clearly indicated that the world was flat! Does that mean that Columbus did not have valuable ideas worth considering?

A survey conducted in 1493 would have turned up significantly different results. The world did not change in those two years but the understanding of the public certainly did!

Research can help explain what happened in the past but it always presents old information. Further, what research reveals is limited by the level of understanding of the people involved the study as well as by the level of understanding of the people interpreting the results.

At one point in history, the popular thinking was that the sun, stars and planets revolved around the earth. It made sense to the people who were interpreting what they saw in the heavens but came from a flawed understanding of what they were seeing. That flawed understanding was "proven" by the "scientific research" of the day but that did not make the conclusions of that research valid

To survive and prosper, you need to be less concerned about where you have been and more focused on where you are going – to be ahead of the pack rather than behind it.

This means there is a premium that comes from listening to those with vision . . . and vision will never be (**can** never be) supported by research except perhaps well after the fact.

Choose your visionaries with care but look ahead, not backward.

40

A Message of Hope From the Field

Here is a message which I share with the permission of the sender. I think it can give us all a few things to think about.

* * * * *

I met you, I believe, last summer at a seminar you did at Campbell's Resort in Chelan, WA. My name is Jerry and I provide excellent customer service on behalf of Campbell's dining room. I wanted to take a moment to let you know how things have been going.

To this day, I practice techniques I learned from you that afternoon and never make less than 18% gratuity. No exaggeration. No need to.

I practice three things: the guest(s) I'm attending to get my undivided attention, eye-contact, and the time I spend at their table, they are the most important reality going. And I smile. Those three habits create the most satisfying win-win situations ($) the position of waiter can offer.

I also consistently do the little things you taught

85

me like including a piece of fresh bread wrapped in cellophane, a pat of butter, included in the leftovers they take along. I also add a fresh baked potato and throw on a fresh garnish if time (and the chef) permits.

I've received written commendations and repeat customers who ask for me. I thought you might like to know that. Thank you again for your time last summer.

Sincerely,
Jerry Wares

I have to tell you briefly my experience of meeting Jerry Wares:

I was first at Campbell's Resort to do a series of seminars for the managers and staff two years ago. I arrived the night before the programs and went down to dinner. Jerry was my waiter.

He was **not** having a good night – he was deep in "the weeds," his timing was off, he was not having a good time and his tables were not having fun, either. It was a situation that was just painful to be a part of!

When he walked into the seminar the next morning, Jerry recognized me. (It was probably not a big thrill for him at that point!) I asked how his evening had gone and he just rolled his eyes. "It was just terrible," he said. "10%, 12% – a real disaster!"

We talked about a number of things at the seminar, including the idea of presence – keeping your mind free from distractions when you are dealing with others.

I saw Jerry later that evening and he was cruising! He had a big grin on his face and his tables were all smiles as well. I caught him by the register and asked him how it was going.

He was excited! He said, "I just got a $25 tip on a $77 check! I have been averaging 25-30% all night!" I asked what he was doing differently and he said, "I am just trying to be *at* the table when I am at the table."

The "Jerry story" has always been a favorite of mine although I have not talked with him since that day. His recent message is very gratifying, of course, but I do not share his note as a testimonial to my seminars (well, at least not *entirely* for that reason!)

What struck me first about Jerry's note was the way he described what he does for a living. I wonder how many servers would say that their job is to "provide excellent customer service on behalf of _____ ." They might mention the service part, but his use of the word *excellent* struck me.

The other point I noticed was that many of the "techniques" he attributes to my seminar were not specific ideas I discussed – they are creations of his own understanding of the principles I introduced and his desire to give his guests a memorable experience. In other words, he had internalized the ideas and now they are entirely his own. This is very exciting to see!

Our education model is outside-in (I am the teacher, I know the stuff and I will beat it into your dense skull until you get it!) There are appropriate places for that type of learning but not when teaching the "soft skills."

Learning people skills is an inside-out process. It happens when trainees see their own answers in their own time and in their own terms. This sort of learning comes more from dialogue than it does from a lecture.

This is actually a much easier (and obviously more effective) way to train than trying to run a classroom session but many managers have a problem with it because it requires they let go of the need to be the source of all information in the organization.

When you are confident enough to let your staff be great . . . on their own terms . . . you will help create a crew of people just like Jerry Wares. I hope you can be so lucky!

41
Watch Yourself

The greatest threat to keeping good staff and managers may not come from the restaurant down the street.

As the rest of the world discovers that service is where it is at – and as they increasingly find that few people in the workforce seem to display a service ethic – it won't be long before they start luring away your best and brightest talent with promises of more money, better benefits and more reasonable work hours. Many are doing it already.

The best defense is a good offense. We must start competing on an entirely new level – the human level – if we hope to be able to grow and prosper in the future.

42

The Making of a Workaholic

Why do so many hospitality managers seem to sacrifice their families and spend endless hours on the job?

Think about this: our industry, while physically demanding, is a source of immediate feedback, usually positive.

Guests pull you aside and thank you for making their experience special. You deal with people who are expecting to have a good time and appreciative of what you do for them.

I know there are some days from Hell, but confess that you love the strokes you get most of the time!

This is a great climate to hang out in and there is always work to do, so it is easy to spend hours on the job.

But while you are on the job being reinforced, the family is at home without you.

When you get home, you get hit with whining kids, a grouchy mate who doesn't know who you are anymore, a long list of projects around the house that need to be done right away – in short, a major hassle.

So consciously or subconsciously, you find yourself spending more time on the job because that is where you are recognized and appreciated.

The more time you stay at work, the worse things become at home and the faster things spiral out of control.

I don't have an easy answer, I just raise the point to see if the pattern looks familiar. If it does, at least you can start to do something about it.

43

The Problem with Higher Checks

Guest expectations rise with the check average, but they rise faster!

This means that a two-dollar increase in the average check may bring a four-dollar increase in the expectations of your guests.

You may be able to get the extra two bucks, but if you cannot deliver the extra $4 worth of experience, you risk alienating your guests.

Be sure you don't upsell yourself down the river!

44

Better than You Have to Be

I recently returned from two weeks in Ireland — both north and the south — where I conducted training programs for several groups who had found me on the Internet. The question that repeatedly came up was, "What do you think of the restaurants in Ireland?"

What I noticed was that the restaurants were only as good as they had to be to stay in business. Perhaps it was lack of strong competition or lack of a model for what was possible. Whatever the case, I had many good meals that could easily have been great meals if a few small points had been addressed.

It occurs to me that it is really no different in our country. Good enough seems to be good enough until some new competition forces operators to raise their food and service to a higher level. I know that everyone is doing the best they can at the moment, but doing the best you can is materially different from being better than you have to be. Why settle for good if you can be great?

Is it a waste of money to be better than you have to be — to do more than is really necessary to give people an unforgettable time? Ask your guests!

45

Do You Have a Martian?

A colleague of mine had what must be the all-time great job. He worked for a regional family restaurant chain and his official title was "Martian." His job was to wander around the units like he had just arrived from another planet and ask questions that might occur to an alien. "Why do you do that?" "What is the reason for _____?" "What's this all about?"

The purpose of this innocent inquiry was to flag the practices and policies that had evolved over time which had no relationship to efficient operations or to making the guest happy.

Do you have a Martian yet? If you did, what might he or she uncover? Do you think you could justify such a position with the savings that would result from eliminating unneeded or unproductive work? Could they likely increase sales by identifying (and resolving) practices that are not guest-friendly?

I suspect the key qualification for a good Martian is that they be removed from the day-to-day of the operation (so they are not invested in how things are presently being done) and that they be insulated from the internal politics of the company (so that they feel free to call 'em like they see 'em.)

Who would be a good Martian for you? Maybe a retired executive in your area would enjoy keeping a hand in the game by wandering around your organization in an alien-like fashion, perhaps in exchange for meals. Someone from the corporate office who doesn't normally spend time "in the field" could be effective if the politics could be kept at bay.

Interestingly, you may find that a new hire at the end of his or her first day of work makes a good short term Martian because their eyes are still fresh. They have only their common sense with which to evaluate what they see going on and are being told.

In the end, the key to a program like this is a real commitment on the part of senior management to consider what the Martian finds and to act on it without regard to whose feelings might be hurt.

If protecting fragile executive egos is more important than moving the company forward, don't waste your time creating a Martian. If no change actually results from having a Martian, the entire program will be a joke.

However, if you have the courage to take a hard look at what you are doing in this way (and to make changes that may be called for) the improvement may truly be "out of this world!"

46

Who Dat?

Is it possible for patrons to dine anonymously in your restaurant?

. . . to have a meal where nobody actually acknowledges them as individuals?

. . . to have an experience where they feel processed instead of being personally served?

. . . to dine when it never appears to matter to anyone on the staff whether the guests are there or not?

Sadly, it happens all too often.

The biggest danger in the hospitality business is that we deliver the service but lose the hospitality – the personal caring that makes guests feel glad they came and anxious to return.

Could anyone dine anonymously in your place? You owe it to yourself (and to your guests) to always know the honest answer to that question.

47
Killing Enthusiasm

We deal in a business of perishables. I am sure you have had the pain of tossing out hundreds of dollars worth of product that had spoiled because of poor handling.

We are sensitized to the perishable nature of raw ingredients, but there is a more precious commodity that we often toss away that can be a more devastating loss – the enthusiasm of our staff.

Have you ever had a staff member come to you with an idea . . . and shot them down because you knew it would not work?

Have you ever thought an employee was "stupid" because their way of seeing things didn't match your own ideas of right and wrong?

Have you ever resisted ideas from your staff because you didn't think of them first?

Do you think the manager's job is to have all the answers?

(Reflect on these questions before answering. If you

are really feeling brave, ask your staff if they have ever observed these behaviors in you.)

If you can answer "yes" to any of these, you are probably guilty of killing enthusiasm.

When it happens, your operation loses, your bottom line loses . . . and you frequently lose a good worker along with it. Can you afford any of these costs?

I previously suggested that the real job of management is not to run the joint, but rather to teach the **staff** how to run the joint! Your job as a coach is to develop the talent of your players, not to prove what a great talent you are yourself.

When someone on your crew gets excited about an idea that they think can make things work better, your job is to embrace that enthusiasm and help channel it in a productive direction.

This does not mean that every idea that comes along is workable, but you will get farther by encouraging their excitement than you will by bursting their bubble.

The valuable commodity is enthusiasm itself, not necessarily the idea they are enthused about.

Whenever you can, give them an opportunity to try their ideas out. If the notion is truly unworkable, they will find out when it doesn't work . . . and they will have learned something. But you might be surprised at how many times they can make something work where you couldn't.

People are more invested in their own ideas than they are in someone else's. You got to where you are today because of all your "great experience," most of which is probably derived from lessons learned in past disasters!

If you do not give your staff the ability and support to test their ideas – on their own, without a net – they will never find out how good they are.

The more you help your staff discover their own unique excellence, the more you can harness their enthusiasm and use it to the good of your operation, the less time you will have to spend on the job, and the more profit you will see.

Never kill enthusiasm. It is your most perishable commodity.

48

Want to Build Sales?

The way to move product is to produce items that are exciting, hire people who can get excited and educate them about what they have to work with.

People love to know things that other people don't know.

When you educate your staff about your food and wines, they will – naturally and enthusiastically – pass that information along to your guests.

There is no word -of-mouth without something to talk about.

49
What is Your Job?

Position descriptions are like a road map to your organization. Properly constructed, they help workers to better understand the game you are asking them to play. Labor litigation also provides real incentives for operators to document the content of each position.

The problem with most job descriptions is that they are little more than lists of activities.

Several times, I worked in operations with activity-based job descriptions. Occasionally I had to conduct a performance appraisal for a worker who was not meeting my standards.

They invariably defended their performance by showing how they had performed every task on their job description. This is akin to claiming to be the world's greatest lover by virtue of having memorized the manual. It is also about as effective!

Why not just define positions in terms of *results* instead of *activities?* Defining results allows people to interpret their jobs in a way that works for them. The immediate advantage is increased productivity, enhanced guest service, improved morale, reduced

101

turnover . . . and more constructive performance appraisals!

A results-based position description has four sections which should be self-explanatory:

Position Summary - a succinct statement of the reason the position exists at all!

Essential Professional Functions - those activities required in the successful performance of the position.

Results Upon Which Performance is Evaluated - the results by which successful performance will be measured.

Qualification Standards - the basic physical requirements of the position in compliance with ADA guidelines.

Position descriptions do not have to be static documents. A colleague of mine opened a new restaurant and used position descriptions as an integral part of his staff training. He spent several days with his new staff discussing the critical results by which they would evaluate each position. They also agreed on the means by which they could tell if they were achieving those results. "I was gratified to discover that my staff had standards that equaled or exceeded my own," he reported.

This article was taken from the book, *The Foolproof Foodservice Selection System,* copyright © 1993 by John Wiley & Sons, Inc. For an example of a results-based position description, just send a self-addressed, stamped envelope and I'll get one off to you.

50

Managing Costs vs. Cutting Costs

I was speaking at the Annual GM Conference for Fresh Choice Restaurants and one of the topics of discussion was the difference between cutting costs and managing costs. It occurred to me that we need to be sure that our staff truly understands the difference.

Less is not more. We must spend the money where we mean to spend the money in order to provide full value to the guest. If we fail to do this, we are just cutting our own throats.

For example, I know of one chef whose response to continual pressure to reduce food cost was to only put one strip of bacon on a sandwich that called for two strips (an unfortunate move in light of the fact that there was a full color picture of the item on the wall of the dining room clearly showing two strips of bacon.)

He honestly thought he was helping, but a guest became so incensed at being "ripped off" that he got into an argument with the manager and stormed out, never to return (and likely to tell all his friends of the incident.) 'Nuff said?

103

51

Your Restaurant is Boring . . .

Your restaurant is boring . . .

. . . if you haven't made changes in your menu in the last two years (price increases don't count)

. . . if you haven't updated your decor in the last five years

. . . if you do not provide continual education for your more experienced workers

. . . if you are only as good as you need to be to stay competitive

. . . if you wait until someone else has proved an idea will work before trying it

. . . if you have not had some spectacular failures in the last three months

. . . if you are the only one in the operation authorized to make a major decision

. . . if you regularly lose talented staff

. . . if you do not visit restaurants outside your market area and find new ideas to adapt

. . . if you never run special promotions or food festivals to break up the routine

. . . if you (and your staff) do not know the names of your regular guests

. . . if you do not receive requests from guests to have specific staff members serve them

. . . if you are regularly working more than 60 hours a week

. . . if you – or your staff – are not having any fun!

Boring restaurants can't compete. Stop it!

You may not agree with all these ideas, but they might be worth pondering.

52

Staff Benefits Revisited

Karen Cooley of Chez Pierre in Tallahassee, Florida pointed out that many of the most attractive (to her staff) benefits cost little or nothing at all!

She has arranged for free checking accounts for her staff at her bank, use of her corporate membership at the local health club (the trendy one that her staff really wants to belong to!), a discount on dry cleaning and dining benefits at the restaurant.

With some thought and a bit of leg-work, I'm sure this list could be expanded even more.

The point of bringing this up is that when you consider benefits, don't limit your thinking to health insurance and 401(k) ideas.

These are good ideas that many would find beneficial but they may not have the same degree of importance to your staff, particularly if you employ younger workers.

53
More Tips for Tips

Here are a few additions to the ideas in my book, *50 Tips to Improve Your Tips.* Kick them around with your service staff and see what happens.

Look at people when you talk to them or serve them anything

This seems almost too basic, but notice how often a server will fail to make eye contact or have their attention elsewhere when serving.

When this happens, it causes guests to trust you less. They are less likely to believe what you tell them or to take your recommendations which can cost you sales (and tips!)

Lack of personal connection when serving makes the food seem less impressive (and that won't help your income either!)

Watch faces as well as tables

You have to watch the tabletop so you will know where the guests are in the meal and what they might need, but that is only part of the job. Watch faces as well.

It will help assure that you notice the guests who are trying to get your attention and will let you see if they are enjoying the meal. If you catch any hint that all is not well, step in and make it right.

Never talk to a table while you are moving

If you talk while you are moving, the message you deliver is, "I've got something happening right now that is more pressing than you are." It will not make the guest feel well-served or eager to leave a good tip.

Go to the table, STOP, make eye contact, say what you have to say and move on. It doesn't take any more time and you will see the results where it counts.

Present the plate

Your food is special, or at least should be treated that way. (It is certainly special to the guest who is about to eat it!) Just plunking a plate down is a disrespectful way to handle the food.

Presenting the plate just means that you PLACE the plate on the table with care, the entree in the six o'clock spot. This is also a natural time to tell the guest something memorable about the item.

There is no word-of-mouth without something to talk about.

54
What's Your Occupancy?

Is that a strange question? Think about a 120-seat restaurant serving lunch and dinner from 11:00am until 10:00pm. On an average day, they do 200 lunches and 200 dinners. Pretty good, right?

Let's look at it again from the aspect of occupancy. What percentage of time is there a guest actually sitting in each chair in the dining room?

If we say the average lunch patron takes 45 minutes to eat, those 200 lunches represent 150 seat-hours (200 meals at ¾ hour each.) If the typical evening meal lasts 90 minutes, the 200 dinners equate to 300 seat-hours (200 meals at 1½ hours each.)

So the restaurant has a total of 500 seat-hours of occupancy.

Now if you figure that the total available supply of seats is 1320 seat-hours (120 seats x 11 hours a day of operation), their occupancy is just under 38%. The restaurant, busy as it is, has unused capacity – time when seats are sitting empty.

I do not mean to suggest that 400 meals a day is some sort of failure in a 120-seat restaurant, but I think many operators would look at the pace of their lunch and dinner business and feel they are running pretty close to capacity. I mean, doing nearly two turns at lunch is quite decent!

But tracking occupancy will show how much room there is for improvement and that knowledge should start your marketing wheels turning to find a way to fill those empty hours.

55

Don't Wash Dishes During the Rush!

Here is another strange idea that may be worth some reflection. If Job One is to make the guest happy, why would we wash dishes in the middle of the rush? Washing dishes doesn't make the guest happy.

(Having a sufficient supply of clean dishes does, but that is not necessarily the same thing!)

In most operations there is no real reason, other than force of habit, why dishes have to be washed during the rush. All it takes is to invest in some additional china, more bus tubs and a few racks.

(Buying equipment is always cheaper than buying labor!)

During the rush, load the racks with tubs of soiled serviceware and pack the dishroom full. When you are over the hump and the pace of business slows, assign two or three people to the dishroom. Wash all the dishes in an hour or so and get on with preparation of the next meal!

This approach can work for most operators,

although high-volume operations and those with tiny dish-rooms may still have to wash during the meal to keep up with the demands of business.

In this situation, workers could work part of their shift on the line and part in the dishroom. A rotation like this would provide cross-training and create a more meaningful job.

I called these folks Assistant Production Managers. Because the job content is greater, the position of Assistant Production Manager merits a higher wage than a dishwasher. The job also requires a different motivation in the applicant.

When the entry level kitchen position is Assistant Production Manager, it will automatically demand more motivated applicants. At the same time, the job will be less attractive to people who are just looking for a few dollars before moving on.

This material was taken from my book, **The Foolproof Foodservice Selection System,** copyright © 1993 by John Wiley & Sons. If you would like a lengthier discussion of this idea, send me a self-addressed, stamped envelope and I'll get it off to you.

56

Sound Familiar?

This amazing bit of trivia concerns experiments in shaping behavior in apes.

Now I doubt that you will be training many primates (although some days it may seem like it!), but see if there is anything in here that strikes a chord:

Start with a cage containing five apes. In the cage, hang a banana on a string and put stairs under it. Before long, an ape will go to the stairs and climb toward the banana. As soon as the ape touches the stairs, spray all of the apes with cold water.

After a while, another ape makes an attempt with the same result – all of the apes are sprayed with cold water. Soon, all the apes realize that if any of them approaches the stairs, all of them will be sprayed with cold water!

Turn off the cold water. Later, if any other ape tries to climb the stairs, the remaining apes will stop him, even though no cold water is sprayed on them.

Now, remove one ape from the cage and replace it with a new one. The new ape sees the banana and tries to climb the stairs. To his horror, all of the

113

other apes attack him. After another attempt and attack, he knows that if he tries to climb the stairs, he will be assaulted.

Next, remove another of the original five apes and replace it with a new one. The newcomer goes to the stairs and is attacked. The previous newcomer will take part in the punishment with enthusiasm. Again, replace a third original ape with a new one. The new one makes it to the stairs and is attacked as well.

Two of the four apes that beat him have no idea why they were not permitted to climb the stairs, or why they are participating in the beating of the newest ape.

After replacing the fourth and fifth original apes, all the apes which have been sprayed with cold water will be gone, yet none of the apes will ever approach the stairs again.

Why not? "Because that's the way it's always been done around here!"

What behavior exists around your place that is no longer supported by either necessity or the expressed desires of management? Where such behavior exists, what do you plan to do about it?

This article was included in my book, *There's GOT to Be an Easier Way to Run a Business,* copyright ©1999 by Hospitality Masters Press.

57

Got a Lemon?
Make Lemonade!

When your next big emergency (fire, food poisoning and such) comes up, make it into a PR opportunity rather than a PR disaster by turning the event into a "how a small business is coping with a major disaster" story rather than having it be an epitaph.

You have to do your thinking beforehand, however. Make friends with key people in your local media, keep in touch with them on a regular basis, develop a plan in the event of a disaster and keep your contact file readily available.

If "the big one" hits you, call the media as soon as possible and give them the alternative angle on the story. Use your specific case as the primary example and broaden the scope enough to provide a hook (and keep it from looking like a fluff piece.)

Did you have a reported case of foodborne illness? Talk about the number of food-related illnesses reported in your area in the last year, noting what a small percentage occurred in public restaurants.

Then talk about how you tracked down the problem, the safeguards that are or were put in

115

place and how the consumer can guard against this sort of problem at home.

Had a fire? Talk about how your guests rallied to your cause, the outpouring of help and goodwill from the community, the history of the restaurant, your struggles to make a small business successful, your awards and honors over the years, how you plan to pull yourself out of the ashes, and the like.

Whatever you do, initiate the action yourself. Do not sit quietly hoping that it will all blow over (it won't!)

But don't waste any time feeling sorry for yourself . . . and don't miss the chance to gain free media space.

Get busy! It will also keep you from becoming reactive and help to put a positive spin on what could otherwise be a negative situation.

58

Get the Kids Involved

While in Tampa recently, a group of us went to dinner at Tuscan Oven, a country Italian restaurant (wood-fired oven, display cooking – great place!)

One of the guys brought his family along, including his 5-year-old son who, naturally, wanted a pizza. The waitress brought the rolled out dough, sauce, cheese and pepperoni . . . and the child made his own pizza right at the table!

The staff took it back to the oven and the child watched as they baked it for him. Talk about thrilled! He even insisted on taking home all of the leftovers of HIS PIZZA!

How can you adapt this idea?

59

What Did You Learn From Your Staff Today?

I often pose this question to operators in my seminars and it is worth bringing up again here. It is a reminder that if you do not have a fresh answer to this question every day, you are not listening.

If you are not listening, you are not learning. If you are not learning, you are not growing. If you are not growing, you will waste away.

I recently asked this question of the people who attended one of my seminars and received the following replies. I thought they might offer a few insights.

I had this exchange with Grant Webb who owns East Side Mario's in Ottawa, Canada:

I learned several things:

1) One of my newer but weaker staff is great at suggesting side salads as an add-on at lunch time. I gave her a pat on the back and told her to keep up the good work.

2) After asking my Patio bartender how things were going, she said that many of the staff were

118

not following opening and closing duty lists on the patio and she finds this very frustrating. I told her that I understood and that I appreciated her feedback.

I will ask some of the other staff the same question in the next few days. I have a feeling that if I ask if they feel the duties were being done right or not, the work will improve on its own – just due to my interest. The best thing is that no discipline is needed to make this happen.

3) I found out a new dishwasher I have teaches developmentally challenged kids how to skate.

4) I asked one of my servers why she was a little off and learned she was very hung over. I thanked her for doing her best and asked if she felt a little silly for punishing herself and her guests with inferior service.

5) I had a chat with another bartender about gardening and kids camps (she has two children). I told her I'd bring some info about a camp I was enrolling my son in.

Thanks for the reminder. I will try to learn more tomorrow.

I responded:
Great news! Amazing what you can learn if you listen. Amazing what you can get done when you don't try to do it all! Please keep me updated as things progress.

119

Grant wrote back:

It is amazing what you can learn when you really listen and it is also amazing what you can see when you actually "watch."

We often find ourselves caught up in the dynamics of this business and forget what our true roles are. My partner and I always used to kid each other that we were the highest paid busboys in the city.

*Not that there is anything wrong in helping out when you are truly needed. The trick is **not** helping out when you are **not** needed. This is something I always knew, but now am finally putting in to practice.*

I think my staff appreciates my feedback and communication more than my running food for them – especially when they don't need it!

You can tap this incredible source of information just by seeing its value. If you listen, you will learn. You might learn something you didn't know. You might get an insight into how another person sees the world. You might pick up an idea that leads to entirely new growth opportunities. But first you have to quiet your mind and really listen. Listen with humility. Listen with curiosity. Listen without judgement. Listen for insights.

What did **you** learn from **your** staff today?

60

Life Goes On
in Many Languages

Wandering among the crowds of tourists in Europe, I heard French, Italian, Spanish, German, Danish, Dutch, Swedish, Russian, English, Japanese, Chinese and several other dialects I didn't recognize.

I was continually reminded that life goes on in many languages – and goes on quite nicely, thank you. While I struggled to make myself understood in French, people seemed to appreciate that I was trying to work in their language. With as fast as our industry is becoming multiethnic, I think there is a lesson here.

We expect our non native-born staff to learn English, but I wonder how much of an effort we are making to learn (at least a bit of) their language?

Communication is communication, regardless of what language it occurs in. How about asking some of your non English-speaking staff to start teaching you some of their language?

Sure, you will butcher the pronunciation and they will all have a good laugh as you struggle with the words, but if you are willing to be uncomfortable in their language, I think they are likely to be more willing to be uncomfortable in English.

We are all just people sharing the same planet. What language we do it in is really not that important in the scheme of things.

It occurred to me that Americans are really cultural lightweights. We have a tendency to think that our way is the best (or worse, the only) way but we don't have near the cultural roots of most other countries on the planet.

I mean, how many other cultures in the world are younger than we are?

I wish everyone could experience this flood of humanity and really see how similar we all are. I think it would make us all a little more tolerant . . . and a lot more humble in the face of those whose cultures predate ours by thousands of years!

When I shared these observations in my Electronic House Call newsletter, I received a number of interesting responses. Here are a few of them.

Paul Rodriguez

I enjoyed your insight on languages. I speak English and Spanish and am trying to learn Italian. I have toured in Europe to find that the average local speaks at least three languages. We should all become multilingual, instead of trying to promote being monolingual in this country. It's good for personal development . . . and it's great for business!

Robert Kausen

Having lived in Europe for four years, I understand what you are saying. To be able to meet people with a sense of deep respect, fascination and eagerness to understanding how they view life turns any trip into a rich experience.

If we remain in the culture we have created in our own minds, then the trip becomes a series of comparisons, judgments, and disappointments. Delighted you are able to do this and have such a grand experience.

Dorothy Wilhelm

Good for you! In my years of living in Thailand and Taiwan, I was so struck by arrogance of the Americans who expected that everyone should speak English. I had the same experience you detail. Although I was never able to speak any other language fluently, I found people delighted when I would at least try.

Luis Fresnedo

In our restaurants in Mexico we joke about languages and by doing so, we create an excellent icebreaker for our foreign customers. For example:

"We don't speak English, but we promise not to laugh at your Spanish"

With a simple sentence like this we encourage our customers to try ordering in Spanish and the staff to speak some English. Everybody has a good time . . . and a good laugh!

123

I agree with you when considering Americans as "cultural lightweights," but I've found most of the American tourists who come to our restaurants are more than willing to learn about and integrate to a different culture.

Nolan Glenn

You make a very good point indeed. Once, I was in a situation where NOT learning a bit of Spanish (the real deal not just the bad words) would have ultimately hindered every aspect of operations. After making a SINCERE effort to learn about their language and culture, I found that the teamwork got a lot better.

I guess my efforts showed others that I was truly interested in them as fellow earthlings and brought mutual respect, trust, enhanced communication and even strong friendships.

Since we all share the desire to be understood and accepted wherever we land in this world, I agree that we should first make the extra effort to learn about others before trying to teach others about us.

So how do *you* approach people of different ethnic backgrounds – as a teacher . . . or as a student?

61
Old Ideas Revisited

"The discipline which makes the soldiers of a free country reliable in battle is not to be gained by harsh or tyrannical treatment. On the contrary, such treatment is far more likely to destroy than to make an army.

"It is possible to impart instruction and to give commands in such manner and such a tone of voice to inspire the soldier no feeling but an intense desire to obey, while the opposite manner and tone of voice cannot fail to excite strong resentment and a desire to disobey.

"The one mode or the other of dealing with subordinates springs from a corresponding spirit in the breast of the commander. He who feels the respect which is due to others cannot fail to inspire in them regard for himself, while he who feels, and hence manifests, disrespect toward others, especially his inferiors, cannot fail to inspire hatred against himself."

> – *Major General John Scholfield*
> *in an address to the West Point Corps of Cadets*
> *August 11, 1897*

62

The Terrible Twos

I get a lot of questions about opening a second unit. Perhaps my thoughts on the subject will help you get ready to expand . . . whether you ever choose to do it or not.

I had an inquiry from someone looking for sources of research to decide where to open a second restaurant. I gave her some ideas and added a comment that prompted the following dialogue:

Q: *You mentioned that opening the second restaurant would be the hardest thing done – more so than the first and all the others following! Would you be kind enough to say why? The first took three years, a lot of money and losses and lessons! We can't imagine why the second would be harder!*

A: Going from one store to two is the hardest jump you make. Two to three, three to thirty is just increasing the size of the game, but one to two is a fundamentally different game.

It is difficult primarily because you can't run two the same way you run one. You are past the point where you can do it all yourself and you go from managing restaurants to managing managers.

You need to have better systems since you will not (necessarily) be on the spot to decide how situations should be handled. In fact, it is usually not that you run #2 and find a manager for #1 . . . you typically end up with two new managers and you get pulled away from the day-to-day of running a restaurant to the business of running the business.

I suggest you get #1 to a point where it can run as well or better without you there before you seriously consider a second unit.

One test is to imagine how it would feel (on both ends of the phone) if you suddenly called the restaurant to say that you have to leave the country for three months and you will not be reachable.

How comfortable would you be with that? How comfortable would your staff be?

When the place can run as well (or better!) without you there, you are ready to consider a second unit. This means that you had better be setting up solid operating systems (and refining them) right now if you ever want to have a prayer of expanding successfully in the future.

Be aware, too, that restaurants are like children. The new child often gets all the attention (and the better decor, equipment, etc.) which creates jealousy and occasional tantrums in the first child.

127

I acknowledge that new projects are more exciting than old ones, but be sure that your first unit doesn't feel abandoned.

In addition to my "gut check" test above, I also advise operators not to let their egos get in the way of their prosperity.

At some level you always know when you are getting in over your head and it is important that you learn to heed that little voice that tells you that you are not the best qualified person to be doing some of the things you are doing.

It is easy to rationalize putting up with your own incompetence by saying that you can't afford anyone else to do it but that is often a cop out. If you really want to do something, you can always find a way to get it done.

So, for example, if you are starting to think about hiring a GM but holding off because of the cost or because you are afraid they will do a better job than you (and make you look bad by comparison) or because you won't have anything to do if you hire a GM, that is a good clue that it's probably time to consider getting more help.

This may be the easiest way to ease into it:

Hire a strong manager to work with you in store #1.

Gradually give this person more and more of the things you have been doing until the new person is essentially running the place without you.

Now you can open store #2 more safely. Get a strong manager there and repeat the process until you are out of the day-to-day in store #2. You are now essentially the director of operations.

When you become more involved with expansion than with operations, either hire an outside operations expert or promote the strongest manager in your system (who should have already trained his replacement.)

The only sure way to expand without killing yourself is to make yourself dispensable first. This is not a bad idea even if you never plan to add more units.

At the very least it will free you up to have a life!

63

Stop Training!

At a CHART Conference (Council of Hotel and Restaurant Trainers), I was impressed to hear that the awareness was shifting from TRAINING people to DEVELOPING people (of which training might be a part.)

The difference is at once simple and profound.

Rather than focusing just on job skills (which is what most training does), we need to be providing what each individual needs to reach his or her fullest potential. This takes us past just job skills to people skills, even life skills.

It signifies an acceptance of each staff member as a total functioning human being, not just a flesh-and-blood machine to be programmed.

It requires a high degree of respect and a deep sense of service.

It suggests we might be interested in having them stick around for a while.

It is a notion worth some reflection.

64

Build Your Network

None of us can know all we need to know to have the life we want – it's too complicated today and there's not enough time to learn it all.

To have the life you want, create a strong network of people who are experts in areas you are not. Then call on this network as needed. That way, you concentrate on doing the things you're here to do and at which you are good and let your network do the rest.

How do you build a network? First, make a list of 50 professions; your list will be different from someone else's list because your activities and strengths are different.

Next, write down at least one name of someone you know and can call on for each of the 50 professions. Finally, note which professions in your list do not have a name and start contacting people who can help you create these new network relationships.

The result? With a strong network your life will get easier, issues will get handled quicker, distractions will be minimized and you will enjoy doing what your life is about.

65

Build Your Database

Marketing guru Tom Feltenstein says that 80% of restaurant business will come from a radius of three miles around your establishment. Are you collecting the names and addresses of all the people who visit your place?

Customers, naturally, are reluctant to provide their names and addresses for use in databases, so you need to use the WIIFM principle (What's In It For Me) if you are going to be successful in gathering names and addresses.

My Aussie colleague, Max Hitchins, also a marketing whiz, owns Billy The Pigs pub in Sydney. Max developed a birthday club to help get past this reluctance. He offers birthday club members $20 of free drinks, free tickets to the latest movie previews and a free voucher for his gaming machines.

Billy's now rates in the top 5% of pubs and taverns in Australia for over the counter bar sales. If you would like a copy of Max's birthday club flyer, send him an email (max@hitchins.com) and include your address. He promises to send one to you. Check him out at www.billythepigs.com.au.

66

Dollars and Sense

Recently I was consulting with a restaurant that had been losing 40 cents on the dollar for a number of years and the owners were tired of writing checks!

The challenge was how to sensitize the staff to the situation without creating mass panic among the troops or revealing figures that were likely to find their way into a feature article in the local paper.

Before I started my first meeting with the staff, I asked them all to write down what percentage of the sales dollar they thought was profit. Then I gave them each $1.00 in change and we started to talk restaurant economics.

The dollar represented a dollar in sales (they understood that) and they also understood there were expenses against it.

Reading from the NRA's Restaurant Industry Operations Report, we started "paying the bills" using median figures for full service restaurants – thirty-five cents for food, thirty cents for labor, five cents for benefits and so on – by dropping the coins into a cup. They were shocked to end up with three cents . . . and that was pre-tax profit!

Then I had them take the money out of the cup and talked about the results that their restaurant was achieving.

We started by paying out 50 cents for food and 50 cents for labor. Then I said, "OK, now we have to pay the rest of the bills – utilities, phone, rent and so forth – so we need another 40 cents. Drop it in the cup. You know that if you don't pay your bills, you won't stay in business."

Their eyes got wide with panic as they tried to figure out where the additional 40 cents was going to come from! I gave the reality of the situation time to settle in before pointing out that when income doesn't cover the expenses, you have to use your own money to stay in business . . . and the owners were tired of it.

They got the message loud and clear and started asking what they could do to help stop the bleeding!

In my experience, unless you educate them to the contrary, most restaurant workers think you make 25-50 cents on the dollar!

By the way, the person who guessed closest to the right answer on the profitability question got the dollar's change from everyone at the meeting . . . and the restaurant's food cost decreased from 53% to 34% in less than six weeks!

67

Expand your Thinking

I recently saw an opinion piece in an industry publication suggesting that because the head chef was so critical to the profitability of the restaurant, managers should be sure they were fully checked-out in that position.

The rationale was that managers needed to be able to run the kitchen so they wouldn't be left hanging when the chef left with all his/her assistants.

The author's view was understandable but I thought it represented a limited frame of reference. For what it may be worth, here is another perspective:

I agree that most managers probably do not spend enough time with the kitchen and that many can be intimidated by their lack of culinary knowledge. However, expecting managers to develop all the talents of their head chef in order to assure success only fosters fear and, in my opinion, is just not realistic.

While the owner should have every position well-covered in the event that key people leave (which they all will do eventually), you can accomplish this most effectively through conscientious staff

135

selection and a consistent staff development program.

It will not happen just by being able to do someone's job for them. (I suspect most managers can probably out-bus the majority of their bussers, but having that skill does not eliminate problems with the bus staff.)

In my experience, managers who are doing what they should be doing – tending to the working climate in the operation, listening to the staff and the guests, providing clear direction and coaching – will not have to worry about the chef leaving with all the crew or suffer the consequences of actions by disgruntled employees.

Managers who are not aware of the impact their own behavior has on the performance of the organization deserve what they get, but becoming a semi-skilled chef or micro managing the kitchen will not assure a pleasant, productive working environment. In fact, it is likely to have exactly the opposite effect.

The manager does not have to know how to do everything better than anyone else – that is why we create organizations. The manager just has to have the ability to recognize when things are on track – or when things are getting off track – and call for the appropriate action at the appropriate time.

Managers don't have to have all the answers, they just need to be able to find the solutions.

In fact, the farther down in the organization the answers come from, the more permanent the results are likely to be and the more the staff will be personally tied into the success of the operation.

In the end, I believe managers should only be doing those things that only they can do.

An increased focus on the functioning of the kitchen (along with the quality and presentation of the food) is probably a good thing in any operation, but it is important to realize that ultimately, a successful restaurant is a human equation.

There are lots of ways to produce success in the hospitality business. Some are just more effortless than others.

68

I Don't Know...

I am continually reminded what a powerful position "I don't know" is.

When you "know," it is easy to stop listening, to stop looking at new possibilities – because you already "know." When this happens, you just look arrogant and pig-headed. (Did you ever work for somebody like this?)

But when a staff member says, "What should I do?" and your first response is, "I don't know. Let's look at this for a second.," it slows your mind down.

You tend to ask more and better questions. You get new and better information. You don't jump to conclusions. You avoid misunderstandings. You tend to consider other points of view. You always learn something new. Ultimately you will do less work because your staff becomes more involved in the process.

To expand on this notion a bit, your goal is actually to get comfortable with the idea of not knowing. In fact, you actually try to "not know" very much. The less you "know," the quieter your mind becomes and the greater the possibilities you will see.

138

The more you become at ease with the idea that you really don't need to know everything (and feel terrific that you don't), the more you will live in this quiet, insightful state. When you think about it, everything you "know" is really just old stuff – it has already happened. Now, past experience has value, but it does not apply to every set of circumstances.

The only real way to know if past experience may be relevant to a present situation is to keep your mind quiet, gather current information and wait for an insight. That process starts with "I don't know" and a healthy curiosity. You see how easily it works?

My colleague, Robert Kausen, puts it this way:

> *"People might find it helpful to think of "I don't know" as the button you press to access deeper creativity.*
>
> *The "Know It All" accesses the data banks for old information. The humility required to go into the "I don't know mode" (the unknown) instantly calls on our deeper creative resources to see something new.*
>
> *(Our egos tend to hate this, but then when did the ego ever come up with anything new and insightful?)*
>
> *It takes some courage initially to get comfortable with the feeling of free-falling in the unknown. Still, the results of spending more and more time in that centered, creative flow of our innate, healthy thinking are well worth it."*

Does this mean that everything you know is wrong?

139

Certainly not. It just suggests that there is always more information than you have. It only makes sense to be sure you have current intelligence on what is actually happening before taking action.

To illustrate, say a bartender comes to you all bent out of shape. "I've got a guy at the bar who is causing a lot of trouble," he snaps. What should I do?" If you slow down long enough to say, "I don't know. What exactly is he doing?" you might find out enough about the situation to be able to make a better suggestion, to ask a more intelligent question . . . or to discover that the bartender already knows how to handle it without you.

For example, asking, "What did you say to him and how did he respond?" will give you a more clear understanding of the situation . . . and keep the responsibility for a solution with the bartender where it belongs.

Not everyone sees things the same way. Your cashier may think the sky is falling when she runs out of tape in the cash register! You would do well to ask more questions before you have a knee jerk reaction and call for a particular course of action.

(By the way, "I don't know" is not the best response in every situation. If the building is on fire, the appropriate response is to tell everyone to leave the building immediately!)

140

When I initiated this discussion of "I don't know" in my e-mail newsletter, I received a number of great responses. Here are several which shed even more light on this notion:

Paula

This is a very important lesson to learn. Many people don't think it's OK to say "I don't know". They think people want an answer, even if they have to make one up. However, I find that saying it does slow you down and allow you to think a little more clearly.

Several years ago I went through a personal transformation, realizing I didn't have to be perfect or know it all. I started saying "I don't know" more and more. It really did liberate me from having to be all-knowing. I don't always remember to use this technique, but I do find it helpful.

Vince

"I don't know" happens to be one of my favorite answers. You really nailed this one! Not only have I worked for people like that, I have had too many employees like that. It takes a long time to get people to understand that it's OK to say "I don't know" when that's the truth.

Sometimes "I don't know" is the right answer. I'm often surprised at how smart and self-confident people can sound when they answer a question with "I don't know" and how shallow and insecure they seem when they try to bluff an answer.

141

Gene

Thanks for the comment on staff bringing questions without solutions or recommendations. They assume that, "Gene will know the answer, let's ask him" without their doing any soul-searching or research. For some of my staff, it is an easy way to get their work done . . . get someone else to do it.

Sometimes I fall into the trap by coming up with an answer without first asking, "What do you think?" It is always assumed the Boss knows so they just ask – and sometimes the Boss thinks he should know so he responds – with an answer that may be less than perfect. Not good, overall.

By admitting you do not know the answer, it takes the pressure of time and accountability away. Sure, I know many answers but not all of them . . . and I shouldn't even be expected to know all of them, right?

Remember, your job is not to **have** the answers, just to be able to **find** the answers – and the best answers often come from other people . . . if you give them the opportunity.

(Note: In my experience, the more certain you are that you are "right," the more likely it is that you are totally off base! At the least, the odds are great that insisting on your opinion at that point will not give you the results you want.)

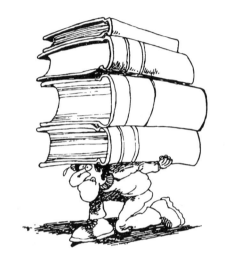

Appendix

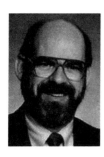

Bill Marvin
The Restaurant Doctor™

Bill Marvin works with companies that want to get more done with less effort and with managers who want to get their lives back! He founded Effortless, Inc., a management research/education company and Prototype Restaurants, a hospitality consulting group.

Bill started his working life at the age of 14, washing dishes (by hand!) in a small restaurant on Cape Cod and went on to earn a degree in Hotel Administration from Cornell University. A veteran of the hospitality industry, Bill has managed hotels, institutions and clubs and owned full service restaurants.

He has had the keys in his hand, his name on the loans and the payrolls to meet. His professional curiosity and practical experience enable him to grasp (and teach) the human factors common to the growth and success of every type of service-oriented enterprise.

He is a member of the Council of Hotel and Restaurant Trainers and the National Speakers Association. He has achieved all major professional certifications in the foodservice industry. He is a prolific author and writes regular columns in the trade magazines of several industries.

In addition to a limited private consulting practice, he logs over 150,000 miles annually delivering corporate keynote addresses and conducting staff and management training programs in the US, Canada, Europe and the Pacific Rim.

EFFORTLESS, INC.
PO Box 280 · Gig Harbor, WA 98335-0280 USA
Toll-free in North America:
Voice: (800) 767-1055 · Fax: (888) 767-1055
Local or outside North America:
Voice: (253) 858-9255 · Fax: (253) 851-6887
e-mail: bill@restaurantdoctor.com
www.restaurantdoctor.com

Reading and Resources

Here is a current summary of materials and services available from Bill Marvin and Effortless, Inc.

Books and Materials

Restaurant Basics: Why Guests Don't Come Back and What You Can Do About It, 1992, John Wiley & Sons

The Foolproof Foodservice Selection System: The Complete Manual for Creating a Quality Staff, 1993, John Wiley & Sons

From Turnover to Teamwork: How to Build and Retain a Customer-Oriented Foodservice Staff, 1994, John Wiley & Sons

50 Tips to Improve Your Tips: The Service Pro's Guide to Delighting Diners, 1995, Hospitality Masters Press

Guest-Based Marketing: How to Gain Foodservice Volume Without Losing Your Shirt, 1997, John Wiley & Sons

50 Proven Ways to Build Restaurant Sales & Profit, 1997, Hospitality Masters Press (editor and contributing author)

Cashing In On Complaints: Turning Disappointed Diners Into Gold, 1997, Hospitality Masters Press

50 Proven Ways to Enhance Guest Service, 1998, Hospitality Masters Press (editor and contributing author)

50 Proven Ways to Build More Profitable Menus, 1998, Hospitality Masters Press (editor and contributing author)

There's GOT to Be an Easier Way to Run a Business, 1999, Hospitality Masters Press

50 Money-Making Marketing Ideas: Increasing Sales by Improving Repeat Patronage, 2000, Hospitality Masters Press

More Restaurant Basics: Why Guests Don't Come Back and What You Can Do About It, 2000, Hospitality Masters Press

Bill also offers audio and video training programs, manuals and computer text files . . . and the list grows steadily. For a current catalog and price list, phone (800) 767-1055 or fax your request toll-free to (888) 767-1055. Locally or outside the US and Canada, call (253) 858-9255 or fax (253) 851-6887.

Keynotes and Seminars

Bill Marvin is generally regarded as the most-booked speaker in the hospitality industry and his messages apply equally well to any service-oriented business. No other speaker takes a similar approach to his subjects, especially in the areas of human relations and organizational effectiveness. He is also one of the few conducting training seminars for the hourly staff.

His keynotes and seminars focus on the human dimensions of hospitality, customer service, staff selection and retention. He is also in demand as a facilitator for executive retreats. When it comes to dealing with people or managing an organization, if you have ever thought, "There *has* to be an easier way to do this," schedule a house call from the Restaurant Doctor™ (even if you are not in the hospitality business!)

Consulting Services

Bill's active speaking schedule does not leave much time for private consulting, but he is always open to an interesting offer and accepts one or two projects a year to keep his skills sharp. His expertise is in the areas of concept development/refinement and increasing sales, retention and productivity by enhancing the work climate of the company.

He has recently started one-on-one coaching with executives who want to deepen their understanding of the principles presented in this book to improve their professional effectiveness . . . and get their lives back!

Newsletters

Bill produces "Electronic House Call," a free weekly newsletter sent by e-mail. To be placed on the EHC mailing list, send your name and e-mail address to bill@restaurantdoctor.com.

Bill also produces the bimonthly "Home Remedies" newsletter where the material in this book originally appeared. To receive a free six-month trial subscription, contact Bill by phone, fax or e-mail and request a sign-up form . . . or complete the sign-up form included on the following page.

147

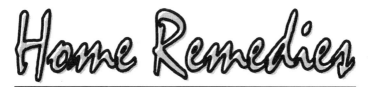

A management journal for service-minded executives

Six months free trial subscription!

Home Remedies is published in January, March, May, July, September and November. The regular subscription price is only $24 a year.

❑ *Yes, sign me up!*

Please start my free trial subscription to Home Remedies newsletter.

PLEASE PRINT CLEARLY

Name _____

Company _____

Address _____

City _____ **State** _____ **Zip** _____

Phone _____ **Fax** _____

e-mail _____

READER INTEREST SURVEY

Information of the type below will not be included in the newsletter mailings – it will be sent ONLY to those who indicate a desire to receive it. Please indicate your level of interest: Yes (Y), No (N) or Maybe (?).

Y N ?

❑ ❑ ❑   *I am interested in knowing when you will be conducting public seminars in my part of the country.*

❑ ❑ ❑   *I am interested in hosting (or co-hosting) an in-house training program for my staff and/or managers.*

❑ ❑ ❑   *I am interested in receiving information on upcoming hospitality industry roundtables.*

❑ ❑ ❑   *I am interested in receiving information on books and materials from Bill Marvin, The Restaurant Doctor™.*

❑ ❑ ❑   *I am interested in receiving information on Bill's seminar and keynote topics.*

Return completed form to:
EFFORTLESS, INC. • PO Box 280 • Gig Harbor, WA 98335
Toll-free Fax: (888) 767-1055